WHAT YOU WILL GET IN THIS BOOK

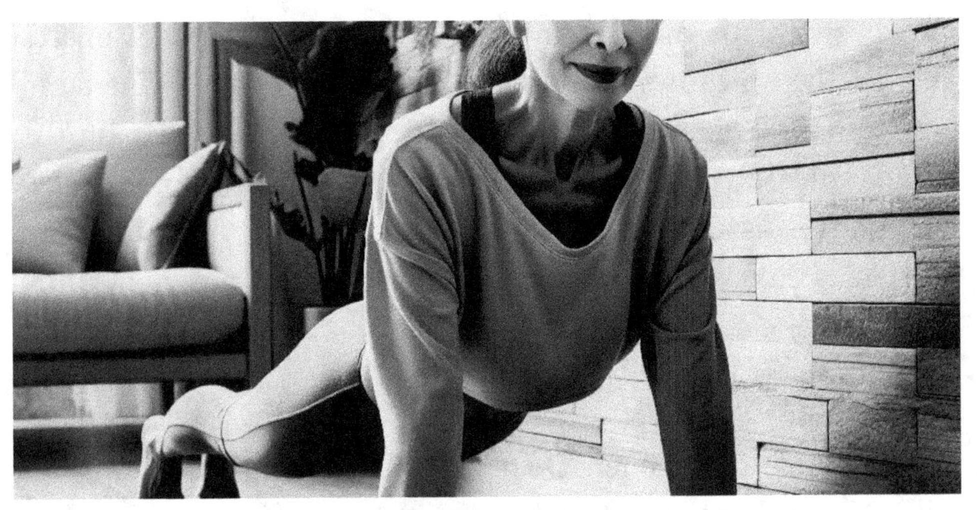

INTRODUCTION

The early sun shines through your window, creating sparkles on the wood floor. You stretch, a subtle soreness reminding you of yesterday's laughter-filled journey, but a greater sense of well-being floods over you. That wasn't always the case. Sixty. The number used to ring like a knell, reminding you of aches, limits, and murmurs of "it's too late."

But then you found wall Pilates. Forget about frightening gyms and bright lighting. This is a symphony performed in your own sun-drenched living room, with the wall serving as your silent companion. There's no expensive equipment, just the sound of your bare feet against cold wood and the quiet murmur of your breath.

Imagine. Your reflection in the mirror moves with you, each movement a brushstroke in a masterpiece of strength and elegance. You find muscles you had no idea were beneath your skin as you waltz with gravity, rejecting its pull inch by inch. There's no grunting or grinding, just the peaceful buzz of resolve and the sun-kissed arc of your leg straining for the sky

However, this is more than simply the physical. It's a protest against the murmurs of aging, a middle finger to stiffness and creaks. Each position is a whispered promise of a pain-free day, a sunrise that infuses your body with new vigor. Anxiety and worry dissolve away in the tranquil folds of your mind, like snowflakes on a warm face. Each inhale is a cleaning wave, and each exhale is a sigh of happiness that echoes throughout your spirit.

Wall Pilates for Women Over 60 is your companion on your trip. We'll explore gentle stretches and mindful movements, as well as breathing methods to put your anxieties to sleep. You'll learn to listen to your body, as it whispers the path to a life full of happiness.

Forget the doubts, sweetheart. This book is a hand extended, an invitation to saunter into a life where you rule supreme. Click here to start this trip together. The sun-warmed wall welcomes your reflection, ready to meet the stronger, happier you.

Remember, age is just a number, and your body is a blank canvas ready to be painted with brilliant colors of power, elegance, and well-being. It's not too late. Open the book, open your heart, and prepare for a new day.

Lets get Started!

CHAPTER 1

Why Wall Pilates?

Forget about banging barbells and frightening mirrors. Wall Pilates does not include seeking "perfection" or pushing your body to its limitations. It's a quiet invitation to dance with your reflection in a sun-drenched space, with your wall serving as a silent partner and your own knowledge as your guide.

But, you may wonder, why is Wall Pilates for bodies engraved with time stories?

Here's why this symphony of power appeals to adult bodies:

- Gentle Yet Powerful: There are no grunts or strains, only the gentle hum of resolve as you fight gravity inch by inch. Wall Pilates sculpts and strengthens using your own body weight and the wall as support, respecting your limits while uncovering latent potential.

- Painless Movement: Stiffness and creaks? We laugh in their faces. Gentle stretches and attentive movements relieve aches and pains, leaving you feeling supple and energized. Each position represents the promise of a pain-free daybreak, a sunrise that fills your body with fresh vitality.

- Balance and Confidence: Are you experiencing wobbly ankles and unsteady steps? Not anymore. Wall Pilates develops your core and improves your balance, restoring your confidence and allowing you to traverse the world with more ease. Imagine the sun on your face, the breeze in your hair, and the confidence that your feet will take you anywhere you choose.

- Bone Health Champion: Osteoporosis has no chance. Wall Pilates routines gently stimulate your bones, increasing density and resilience, and strengthening you from the inside out. Your bones may sing a young melody with the correct care, even though age is just a number.
- Mind-Body Harmony: It's not just about the physical. Wall Pilates is the entrance to your inner sanctuary, a place where tension melts away like snowflakes on a warm cheek. Each inhalation is a cleaning wave, and each exhale is a sigh of happiness that resonates in the quietest corners of your soul. Forget your troubles and cares, and let them go with each soft stroke.

"Why Wall Pilates?" It's a question that your body answers by whispering thanks after each session. It's in the renewed bounce in your stride, the confidence in your eyes, and the satisfaction of regaining your power and elegance. The symphony of well-being echoes from within.

So, open the door to your sun-drenched hideaway, let the wall be your friend, and experience Wall Pilates' transformational power. It's time to rewrite your tale, one delicate motion at a time.

Setting Your Goals

Picture this: Standing tall with your shoulders back and chin raised high. You walk with fresh grace, a symphony of power and confidence reverberating in every step. Aches and pains are no longer the unpleasant soundtrack to your life. This is not a pipe dream; it is the reality that awaits you after you uncover the revolutionary potential of "Wall Pilates for Women Over 60."

However, before you go on this trip, you must first sow the seeds of your change by establishing your goals. Forget boilerplate resolutions that fade faster than fall leaves. We're talking about carving objectives into the foundation of your desire, goals that provide a clear image of the life you want to live.

Do you dream of:

- Say goodbye to that persistent soreness in your lower back. Wall Pilates will help you strengthen your core and improve your posture, making discomfort a distant memory.
- Climbing stairs like a gazelle? Gentle workouts for elderly bodies will leave you feeling powerful and energized, ready to face any challenge.
- Feeling the sun on your face as you briskly stroll along the beach? Improved balance and coordination will allow you to navigate the world with renewed confidence, with each stride demonstrating your strength.
- Trading your joints' creaks and moans for a whisper of painless movement? Gentle stretches and attentive movements can help your body regain its vitality, restoring flexibility and making you feel supple and lively.

But objectives are more than simply wishes; they are plans for action. "Wall Pilates for Women Over 60" can help you set SMART objectives that are specific, measurable, attainable, relevant, and time-bound. We'll help you transform your ambitions into actionable steps, celebrating each milestone along the way.

Remember, it's not about pursuing unachievable goals or pushing yourself to the limit. It's about listening to your body, interpreting its cues, and developing objectives that reflect your own needs and wants.

So, pick your pen, and let's create your future together. What does it look like to be pain-free and graceful? What ambitions would make your heart sing? With each stroke of your pen, you get closer to the vivid song of well-being that lies ahead.

Open the book, open your heart, and welcome a life filled with power, grace, and joy. Your objectives are your compass, and "Wall Pilates for Women Over 60" is your chart. Let us go on this adventure together

Strategies for tracking progress towards physical therapy goals

Tracking progress toward physical therapy objectives is critical for ensuring that people make improvement and stay on track. Here are several techniques to measure progress:

- Document improvements and setbacks. Keep track of your progress and how physical therapy helped to alleviate your discomfort. This might help you stay motivated and realize how far you've come.
- Set SMART goals: Setting specified, measurable, attainable, relevant, and time-bound (SMART) goals will help you stay focused and measure your progress.
- Regular check-ins: Schedule frequent check-ins with your physical therapist to verify you're making progress and change your goals as necessary.
- Tracking your capacity to complete everyday duties or sports-related activities might give useful information on your rehabilitation.

- Monitor your total pain level on a daily basis to track your improvement.
- Keep track of your activity level, since it often increases faster than the pain level reduces.
- Home exercises: Consistently do your recommended home workouts to help you stay motivated and devoted to your rehabilitation.
- Partner up: Find a support system, such as a friend or family member, who can assist hold you accountable for attending physical therapy sessions and sticking to your treatment plan.

Implementing these tactics will allow you to properly track your progress toward physical therapy goals and guarantee that you get the most of your rehabilitation experience.

Understanding your body

Forget murmurs of "too late" and echoes of "used to be." In Wall Pilates for Seniors Over 60: Understanding Your Body, we rewrite the story of aging, converting restrictions into pathways to a more vibrant and empowered you.

Here is where the magic occurs:

- Unmasking Common Concerns: Back discomfort, creaking knees, and unstable balance: aging may hurl these curveballs at us, but we'll figure out how to deal with them. We'll look at the why behind the discomfort, wobble, and stiffness, giving you the knowledge to face them front on and pave the road for pain-free mobility.

- From Limits to Detours: Forget "can't" and say "can-do, with a twist!" We'll show you how constraints aren't dead ends, but rather detours leading to secret routes. Modified workouts, alternate alternatives, and an emphasis on listening to your body's knowledge will serve as your guides as you navigate your particular terrain and find your well-being oasis.

- Bone Building Symphony: Age may be whispering about bone density, but we'll respond with a calm, strengthening symphony. We'll introduce workouts that work with your bones to create a song of power and resilience from inside. Forget frailty; your bones can learn a new, strong melody.

- Emotional Harmony: Aging is more than simply physical; it is also a tango of emotions. We'll address the fears and whispers of doubt that might come with physical changes, and we'll teach you mindfulness practices and gentle movements to calm your mind and align your spirit with your body.

- Your Body and Your Compass: Forget the one-size-fits-all approach. We'll teach you how to listen to your body's unique whispers and grasp the language of aches, moans, and quiet delights. This inner wisdom serves as a compass, guiding you to customize your practice, select activities that connect with you, and confidently chart your path to well-being.

Wall Pilates for Seniors Over 60: is more than simply a book; it's a discussion starter, a mapmaker, and a motivator. It's your dependable friend on the path of redefine what it means to move, feel, and be at any age. So, open the book, your intellect, and your heart to your own body's knowledge. We'll rewrite your tale, one attentive action at a time.

Remember that age is simply a number, and your body is a canvas ready to be painted with the brilliant colors of self-awareness, resilience, and joy. It's time to listen, comprehend, and realize the potential that exists inside. Let's rewrite your tale together.

Embracing the mind-body connection

In your sun-drenched living room, the wall communicates not just encouragement, but also a deep truth: your body and mind are partners in this dance called life. Wall Pilates for Seniors Over 60: Embracing the Mind-Body Connection allows you to take the stage, where movement becomes a symphony and quiet is a refuge.

Forget about the gap between exercise routines and emotional well-being. Weave together the threads of physical activity with inner tranquility to create a tapestry of comprehensive well-being.

Imagine this:

Each quiet breath: a cleaning wave that washes away your worries, leaving you peaceful and balanced.

Each attentive movement is a brushstroke that creates a masterpiece of inner harmony, combining power and calm.

The gentle hum of your concentration: a tune that drowns out the babble of doubt and concern, leaving you feeling anchored and present.

This is not about contortion or Olympic exploits. It is about listening to your body and mind's delicate dialog and reacting with gentle movements and attentive breathing. We will explore strategies such as:

- Guided visualization: Create vivid mental images of serenity, allowing them to sink into your muscles, reducing tension and promoting relaxation.
- Mindful movement is focusing on each stride, stretch, and breath, bringing awareness to the present moment and suppressing mental chatter.
- Positive affirmations: Counter whispers of doubt with calm, uplifting remarks that promote self-esteem and confidence.
- What are the benefits? A melody of wellness:
- Reduced tension and anxiety: With each soothing movement, you will discover calm in your own refuge.
- Improved sleep: Calm your thoughts and lull your body into a deep, peaceful slumber, waking up feeling refreshed and energetic.
- Increased emotional resilience: Develop the inner strength to face life's hardships with grace and acceptance.
- A closer connection to oneself: Listen to your body's whispers, learn its language, and develop a sense of self-worth and respect.

Embracing the Mind-Body Connection" will help you through this journey of comprehensive well-being. It's a whisper in the breeze, an invitation to dance with your reflection in the sunny mirror, and a reminder that you are whole in body, mind, and soul. So, open the book, open your heart, and prepare to live a life full of serenity, power, and joy.

Remember that age is simply a number, and your body is a temple ready to be filled with the song of mindfulness and the light of self-acceptance. It is time to listen, connect, and feel the transformational power of the mind-body symphony. Let's rewrite your tale together.

CHAPTER 2

Building a Strong Foundation

Building a Strong Foundation isn't about pumping iron or chiseling abs. It's all about building a rock-solid core from the inside out, radiating strength, stability, and confidence every step of the way. Forget rickety steps and delicate whispers; this is about creating a fortress of well-being.

Here's what Building a Strong Foundation means to you:

- Goodbye to Wobbly Anxieties: Fear of falls? Not any more! Gentle exercises will strengthen your core and enhance your balance, allowing you to traverse the world with greater elegance and stability.
- Eliminating Back Pain: No more backaches stealing your happiness! We'll sculpt your core muscles, correct your posture, and strengthen your spine to create a natural support system that relieves pains and leaves you feeling flexible and pain-free.
- Climb Stairs with Gazelle-like Ease: Stairs used to be scary obstacles? Forget it! We'll strengthen your leg muscles and increase your flexibility, transforming those stairs into simply stepping stones on your path to a full existence.
- Building Bone Density Like a Rock: Age may whisper about bone loss, but we'll reply with a symphony of mild activities that stimulate your bones, increasing density and toughness. From the inside out, your foundation will grow stronger and more stable.
- Owning Your Strength, One Mindful Movement at a Time: Let go of the need to push yourself beyond your boundaries.

We will help you listen to your body, comprehend its messages, and construct your foundation at your own speed. Every thoughtful action counts, every mild stretch is an accomplishment, and every discomfort alleviated demonstrates your increasing strength

Building a Strong Foundation in the Wall Pilates is about more than simply physical outcomes; it's about changing the way you feel and move. It's all about having confidence, feeling empowered, and embracing your inner strength. So, open the book, open your mind, and listen to your body's whispers. Let us work together to create a strong fortress, one attentive movement at a time.

Remember, age is just a number, and your body is a blank canvas ready to be painted with the brilliant colors of power, resilience, and confidence. It's time to set the groundwork for a life full of possibilities, founded on grace, awareness, and the power of your own will.

Perfect Posture

The ideal posture in wall Pilates for women over 60 is maintaining good alignment and stability while completing exercises against a wall. Here's a concise and straightforward explanation:

- Alignment: Stand with your back to the wall, maintaining your head, shoulders, and hips in contact with it. Your feet should be hip-width apart, a few inches from the wall.
- Core Engagement: To activate your core muscles, gently bring your navel toward your spine. This helps to support and stabilize your lower back.
- Shoulder and Neck: Keep your shoulders down and back, without hunching or rounding.

Keep your neck extended and in a neutral position.

- Knees and Hips: Soften your knees slightly to prevent locking them, and keep your hips, knees, and ankles aligned.
- Breathing: As you complete the exercises, breathe deeply and evenly while keeping your core aligned and engaged.

This position promotes optimal spinal alignment, core strength, and general stability, which is especially good for women over 60 to maintain their musculoskeletal health and mobility

Breathing for Life

Breathing is a vital component of wall Pilates for women over 60, complementing the movements. Some breathing techniques used include

- Diaphragmatic Breathing: Concentrate on deep diaphragmatic breathing, allowing the belly to expand on inhalation and gently constrict on exhalation. This sort of breathing encourages relaxation and engages the deep core muscles.
- Rhythmic breathing: Coordinate your breathing with the actions. Inhale at the first portion of the movement and exhale throughout the effort period. This regular breathing increases the efficiency of the workouts and aids in stability.
- Mindful Breathing: Throughout the exercises, keep your breath steady and regulated. This mindfulness practice improves attention, decreases stress, and strengthens the mind-body connection.

Women over 60 who incorporate these breathing strategies into their wall Pilates practice can enjoy higher oxygenation, stronger core engagement, and a greater sensation of calm and focus.

Core Essentials

Core Essentials is a mild yet effective path to developing a strong, solid core without breaking a sweat. Here's your guide to living a flourishing life, one mindful action at a time:

- Building Your Powerhouse: Your core is more than simply six-pack abs; it serves as the basis for all you accomplish. We'll work on all of the hidden muscles deep within, establishing a natural support system that enhances your balance, posture, and strength.

- Goodbye, Wobbly Anxies: Is your fear of falling causing you to lose joy? Gentle workouts can strengthen your core, making you feel stable and secure on your feet. Navigate the world with renewed elegance, knowing that your inner strength has your back (and everything else!).

- Get Rid of Back Pain: Backaches will no longer be welcome guests. We'll sculpt and strengthen your core muscles, readjust your posture, and make your spine more flexible. Say welcome to pain-free mobility and rediscover the delight of feeling supple.

- Breathe Easier and Move Freer: A strong core is more than simply muscles; it also supports your breathing. We'll show you how to maximize your breathing capacity, allowing you to move freely while infusing your body with life-giving oxygen.

- Mindful Movements, Big Results: Forget the temptation to push yourself.

This is about listening to and honoring your body's whispers. Every gentle stretch and thoughtful movement helps to strengthen your core and improve your overall well-being.

Here is your Action plan:

- Begin with the Wall: Your wall is your silent companion, offering support and stability as you perform mild exercises such as pelvic tilts, wall holds, and core-activating stretches.
- Breathe With Intention: Concentrate on your breathing, linking each inhalation with core engagement and each exhale with tension relief.
- Progress at Your Own Pace: There is no Olympic race here. Listen to your body, adjust routines as required, and applaud every accomplishment, large or little.
- Feel The Difference: As your core improves, you'll notice improved balance, posture, pain-free movement, and an inner sense of confidence.

Remember that your core is the driving force behind every move you take. Core Essentials teaches you how to nurture your powerhouse, unleash its potential, and create a masterpiece of strength, elegance, and well-being on your life's canvas. Open the book, mind, and heart to your body's whispers. Let's work together to construct a core that will set you free.

Gentle Mobilization

Gentle mobilization in the wall Pilates for women over 60 consists of low-impact exercises that increase joint mobility and flexibility. Here's a simple and straightforward explanation with instructions

- Warm-up: To prepare your body for movement, start with a mild warm-up, such as walking in place or performing shoulder rolls.
- Joint Mobilization: Do exercises that mobilize the joints, such as ankle circles, wrist circles, and neck rolls. These exercises assist to increase joint range of motion and reduce stiffness.
- Low-impact exercises: Choose low-impact, joint-friendly activities like leg lifts, arm circles, and wall squats. These exercises develop strength, flexibility, and balance while putting minimal strain on the joints.
- Finish your workout with a mild cool-down, such as stretching or deep breathing, to encourage relaxation and prevent muscular pain.

Here is your action plan:

- Focus on Quality: Slow, deliberate motions are essential. Concentrate on experiencing each stretch, linking your breath to your movement, and acknowledging your body's input.
- Target all areas. We'll work on mild stretches for your neck, shoulders, spine, hips, knees, and ankles, making sure no creaks or groans go undetected.
- Embrace the Wall: Think of your wall as a helpful buddy, providing stability and aid while you experiment with modest mobilizations.
- Celebrate your progress by noticing tiny triumphs such as greater range of motion, less discomfort, and improved balance. Each stride represents your developing independence.

Note, that gentle mobilization is more than just stretching; it is about listening to and nourishing your body's knowledge. Let's move with elegance and ease, one soft stretch at a time

CHAPTER 3

Wall Pilates in Action Beginner Routines

Wall Pilates is a variant on standard Pilates exercises that uses a wall for support and resistance, therefore improving stability, alignment, and strength. Beginner routines in Wall Pilates focus on developing basic abilities while also giving support for people who are new to Pilates or who require assistance with balance and stability.

A typical beginner program may begin with a simple warm-up to move the spine and joints, such as marching in place or doing arm circles. The wall provides a secure barrier for support throughout these motions, enabling participants to concentrate on perfect alignment and technique without the risk of falling.

Exercises frequently use the wall to offer both support and resistance. For example, a newbie may begin with Wall Squats, in which they rest against the wall with their feet hip-distance apart and gradually bend their knees, sliding down the wall into a squat posture. This improves leg strength while simultaneously teaching good squat technique.

Another fundamental exercise is the Wall Roll-Down, in which the participant stands with their back against the wall and gradually articulates their spine, rolling down one vertebra at a time until their hands touch the floor. Then they roll back up to standing, utilizing the wall as support throughout the maneuver. This exercise helps to increase spinal mobility and body awareness.

Beginner routines sometimes include wall push-ups, in which participants stand facing the wall with their hands at shoulder height. They next bend their elbows, drop their chest on the wall, and push back up to their starting position. This workout increases upper-body strength and is more accessible than typical floor push-ups.

These exercises emphasize good breathing methods and conscious movement. Participants are taught to keep their spine neutral and use their core muscles to support their movements. As individuals advance, they may gradually increase the intensity and complexity of the exercises in order to challenge their bodies and improve their Pilates practice.

Wall Angel

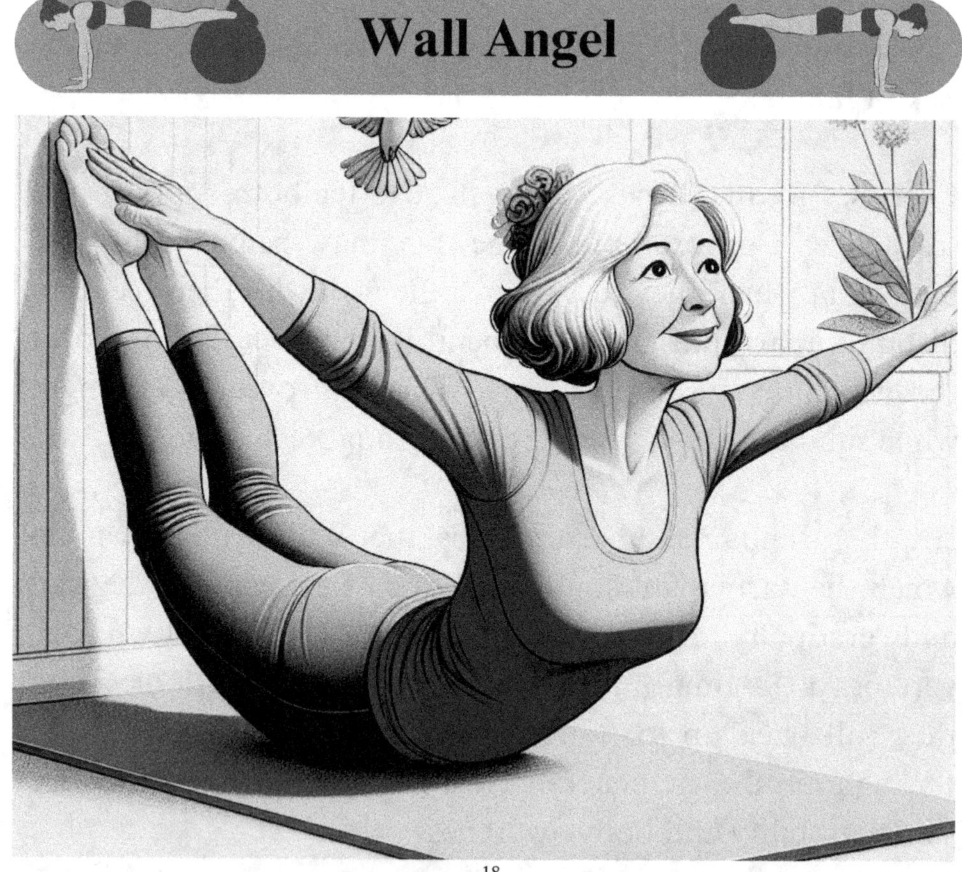

How to Do:

1. To do wall angels, begin by standing with your feet hip-distance apart and your back to the wall. Engage your core muscles to keep your spine neutral throughout the workout. Extend your arms out to the sides at shoulder height, palms facing front, with elbows slightly bent.
2. Next, carefully slide your arms up the wall, maintaining them in contact with the surface at all times, until your hands are over your head. To avoid shrugging, lift your arms while keeping your shoulders down and away from your ears. Once your arms are fully stretched overhead, pause briefly before carefully lowering them back to shoulder height.
3. Maintain proper posture and alignment throughout the action, keeping your lower back pressed against the wall and your chin parallel to the floor. Avoid arching your back or letting your ribs flare out.
4. Wall angels assist to improve posture by strengthening the muscles of the upper back, shoulders, and core, which are essential for maintaining good alignment and spine support. They also improve shoulder mobility and flexibility, lowering the chance of injury and pain.

To get the most out of wall angels, move slowly and with control, focusing on the quality of your movement rather than speed or quantity. Begin with a few repetitions and progressively increase as you gain familiarity with the exercise. Incorporating wall angels into your Pilates exercise will help you establish a solid foundation for improved posture and general body awareness.

Wall leg lifts

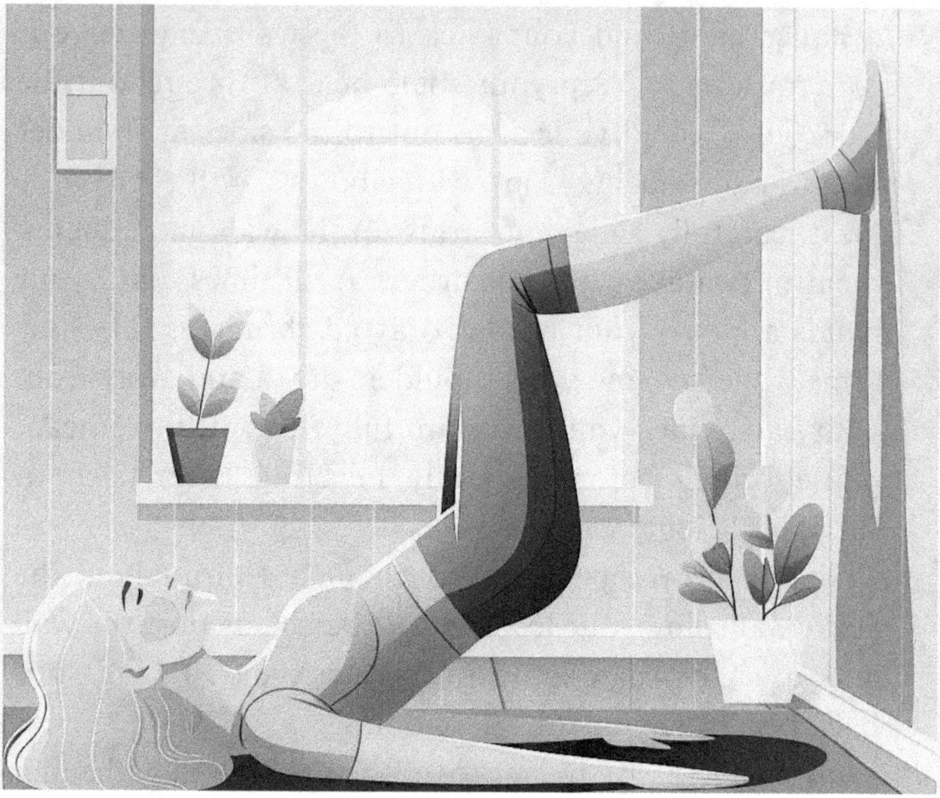

Wall leg lifts are an excellent exercise for developing the lower body muscles, especially the legs and core, while receiving mild assistance from a wall. Here's a simple step-by-step tutorial for completing wall leg lifts:

How to Do:

- Set up: Stand with your side facing a wall, approximately an arm's length away. Place one hand gently on the wall for support and maintain a straight line from your head to your heels.

- Engage your core muscles by pulling your belly button towards your spine.

This engagement helps to support your torso and keep appropriate posture during the activity.

- Position Your Legs: Start with your feet hip width apart. Shift your weight slightly to one leg while keeping both legs straight. The standing leg will serve as the exercise's foundation of support.
- Lift Your Leg: Slowly raise your other leg out to the side, keeping it straight and under control throughout the action. Aim to elevate your leg to hip height or slightly higher, depending on your flexibility and comfort.
- Pause at the Top: When your leg reaches its highest position, take a little moment to focus on stability and balance. Maintain your hips level and prevent leaning or tipping your upper body to one side.
- Lower Your Leg: Controlfully lower your leg back to its initial position. Maintain a smooth and controlled motion, utilizing the muscles of the standing leg to aid in the lowering phase.
- Repeat the action on the opposite side, altering your hand location on the wall as necessary for stability. Alternate between legs for the appropriate number of reps or duration.
- Maintain Proper Alignment: Throughout the workout, keep your body aligned. Maintain a relaxed shoulders, raised chest, and neutral spine. Avoid arching or rounding the lower back.
- Breathe: Keep your breathing steady and regular throughout the activity.

Inhale as you elevate your leg, exhale as you lower it, and keep a comfortable breathing pattern to help you move.

- Adjust Intensity: Depending on your fitness level and comfort, you may make the workout easier or more challenging by modifying the height of your leg lift or the distance from the wall.

Following these step-by-step instructions will allow you to do wall leg lifts successfully, strengthening your lower body muscles while benefiting from the wall's soft support. Gradually increasing the amount of repetitions or adding resistance as you go will help to test your muscles and increase your total lower-body strength.

Sidekicks against the wall

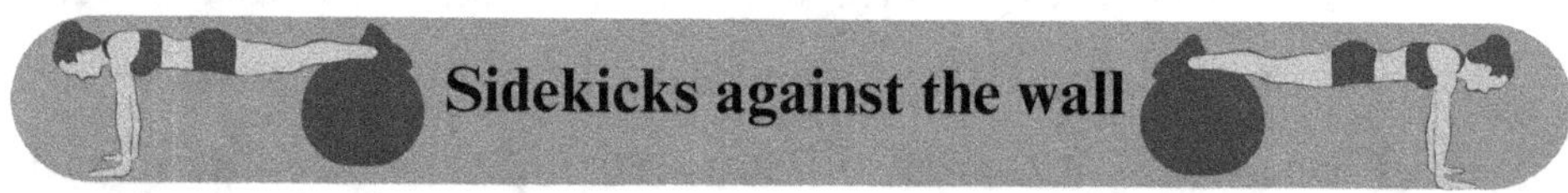

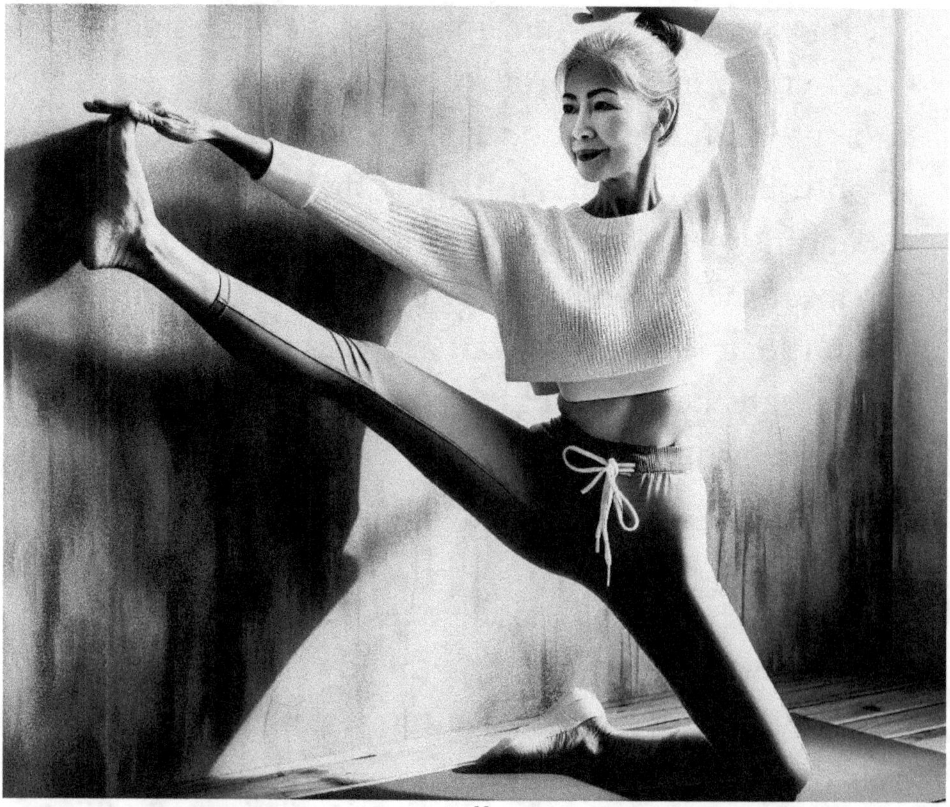

Sidekicks against the wall are an excellent exercise for developing core strength and stability while focusing on leg and hip muscle groups. Here's a step-by-step instruction for doing sidekicks against the wall.

How to Do:

- Set up: Stand with your side facing a wall, approximately an arm's length away. Place one hand lightly on the wall for support while maintaining your arm straight. Maintain a straight line from your head to your heels.
- Engage your core muscles by pulling your belly button towards your spine. This engagement helps to support your torso and keep appropriate posture during the activity.
- Position Your Legs: Start with your feet hip width apart. Shift your weight slightly to one leg while keeping both legs straight. The standing leg will serve as the exercise's foundation of support.
- Lift Your Leg: Slowly raise your other leg straight out to the side, keeping it parallel to the ground and under control throughout the exercise. Aim to elevate your leg to hip height or slightly higher, depending on your flexibility and comfort.
- Point Your Toes: Flex your foot and point your toes towards the wall to activate the leg muscles and form a powerful, straight line from hip to heel.
- Pause at the Top: When your leg reaches its highest position, take a little moment to focus on stability and balance. Maintain your hips level and prevent leaning or tipping your upper body to one side.
- Lower Your Leg: Controlfully lower your leg back to its initial position.

Maintain a smooth and controlled motion, utilizing the muscles of the standing leg to aid in the lowering phase.

- Repeat the action on the opposite side, altering your hand location on the wall as necessary for stability. Alternate between legs for the appropriate number of reps or duration.
- Maintain Proper Alignment: Throughout the workout, keep your body aligned. Maintain a relaxed shoulders, raised chest, and neutral spine. Avoid arching or rounding the lower back.
- Breathe: Keep your breathing steady and regular throughout the activity. Inhale as you elevate your leg, exhale as you lower it, and keep a comfortable breathing pattern to help you move.

By following these step-by-step directions, you may execute sidekicks against the wall to improve core strength and stability while targeting leg and hip muscles. Gradually increasing the amount of repetitions or adding resistance as you develop will help to test your muscles while also improving your overall strength and stability.

Bridge variations

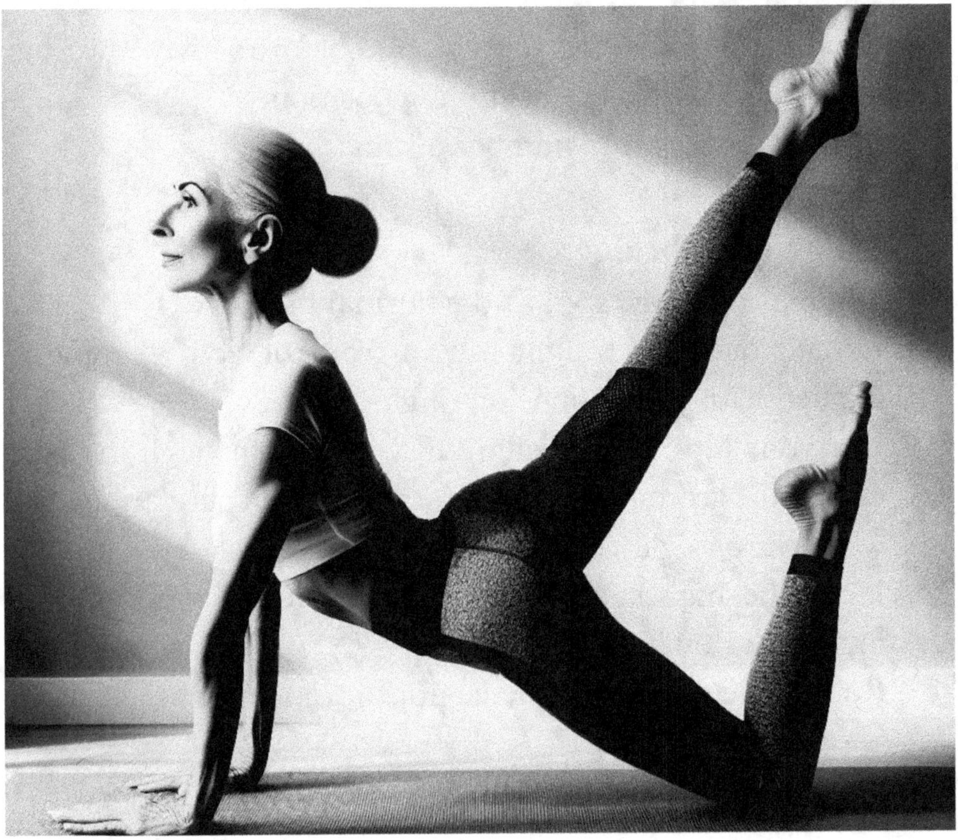

Bridge variants are great for working the glutes and hamstrings, which strengthens the back and increases overall stability. Here's a step-by-step method for performing bridge variations

1. **Standard bridge:**
   - Lie on your back, knees bent, feet flat on the floor, hip-width apart. Your arms should be lying at your sides, palms facing down.
   - Gently drag your belly button towards your spine to engage your core muscles.

- To elevate your hips towards the ceiling, press through your heels and squeeze your glutes at the apex of the exercise.
- Hold the top position for a second before slowly lowering your hips back to the beginning position.
- Repeat the required number of times.

2.   Single-leg bridge:

- Begin at the same spot as the normal bridge.
- Extend one leg straight out in front of you, keeping it aligned with your opposing thigh.
- Lift your hips to the ceiling by pressing through the heel of your grounded foot, focusing on activating the working leg's glutes and hamstrings.
- Hold the highest position briefly before lowering your hips back down.
- Repeat the same side for the appropriate number of times before switching legs.

3.   Bridge and Leg Lift:

- Start in the typical bridge posture, with both feet level on the floor.
- Lift one leg straight up to the ceiling while keeping the other foot firmly on the ground.
- Lift your hips towards the ceiling by pressing through the grounded heel, maintaining stability and working the glutes and hamstrings.
- Hold the highest position briefly before lowering your hips back down.
- Repeat the same side for the appropriate number of times before switching legs.

4.   Bridge with Stability Balls:

- Lie on your back, legs bent, feet resting on a stability ball.
- Use your core muscles to help maintain your spine.
- Lift your hips towards the ceiling by pressing your heels and moving the stability ball towards your body.
- Hold the top posture briefly before slowly lowering your hips and moving the ball away from your body.
- Repeat the appropriate number of times, concentrating on control and stability throughout the action

5.   Bridge with Resistance Bands:

- Place a resistance band slightly above your knees and lie on your back, knees bent and feet flat on the ground.
- To activate the hip abductors, engage your core muscles and squeeze your knees against the resistance band.
- Lift your hips to the ceiling, squeezing your glutes at the height of the motion.
- Hold the top position for a brief while before slowly lowering your hips back to the beginning position.
- Repeat for the appropriate number of repetitions, keeping the resistance band tight throughout the exercise.

Incorporating these bridge variants into your workout will efficiently activate your glutes and hamstrings, strengthening your back and improving overall stability. Begin with the conventional bridge and progressively move to more difficult versions as you gain strength and confidence.

"Every stretch brings you closer to your best self."

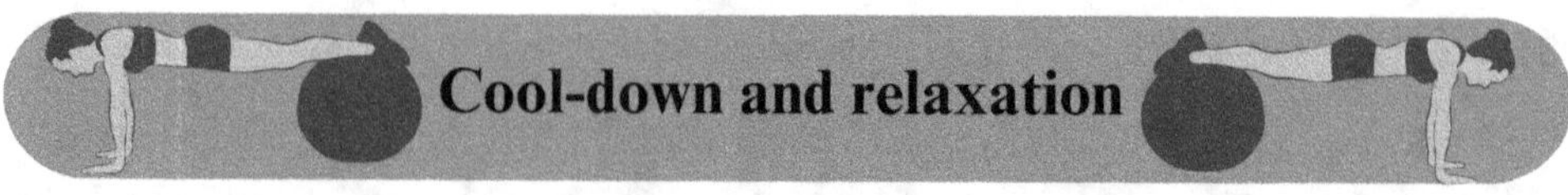

Cooling down and relaxation are key components of every workout regimen, as they serve to reduce muscular tension, enhance healing, and restore body and mind peace. Here's a step-by-step method to unwinding for serenity and healing:

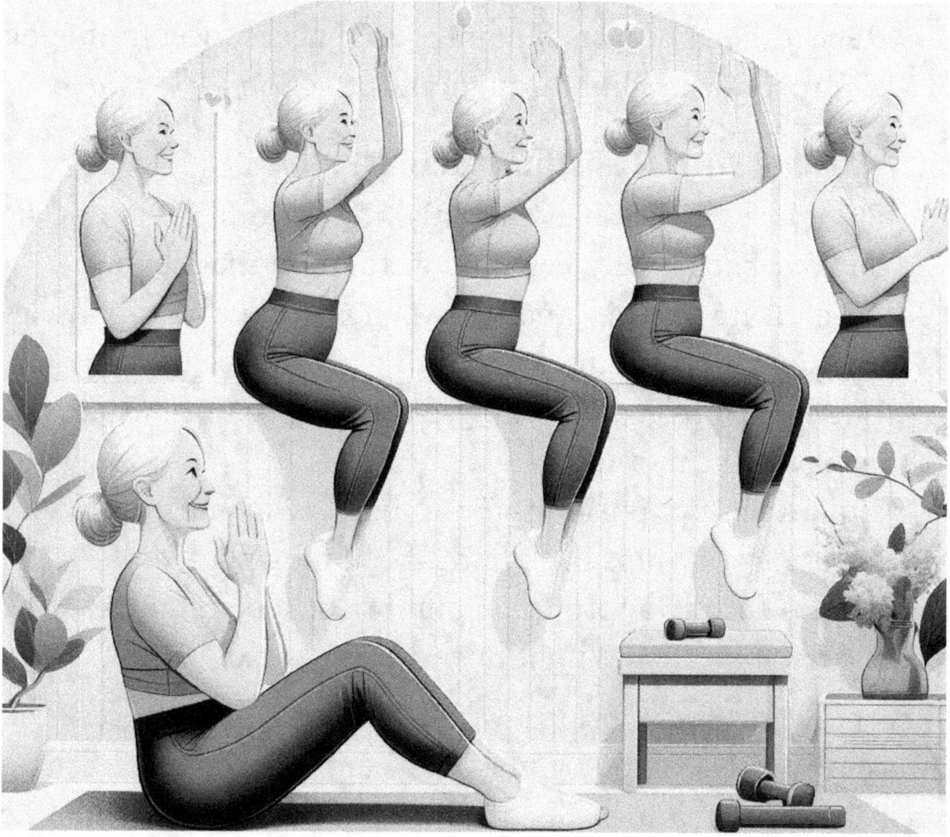

How To DO:

- Deep Breathing: Start by selecting a comfortable sitting or sleeping posture. Close your eyes and take a few calm, deep breaths, in through your nose and out through your mouth. Concentrate on filling your lungs with oxygen and releasing any tension with each breath.

- Gentle Stretching: Do a series of gentle stretches to relieve tension in the muscles engaged throughout your workout. Concentrate on stretching key muscular groups such the legs, hips, back, shoulders, and neck. Hold each stretch for 15-30 seconds, and avoid jumping or pushing beyond your comfort level.
- Foam rolling: Use a foam roller to conduct self-myofascial release on tight or aching muscles. Roll carefully and thoughtfully across each muscle group, pausing at any points of tension or discomfort. Maintain calm breathing during the procedure.
- Mindfulness Meditation: Use mindfulness meditation to clear your thoughts and promote calm. Sit comfortably, eyes closed, and focus your attention on the present moment. Without passing judgment, pay attention to any feelings in your body, noises in your surroundings, or ideas that come to mind. Allow yourself to just be there and watch without responding.
- Progressive muscular relaxation involves releasing tension from head to toe. Begin by tensing and then releasing each muscle group in your body, from your forehead to your toes. Concentrate on the sense of relaxation flowing through each muscle as you eliminate tension.
- Listening to a guided imagery meditation or visualization might help you relax and clear your mind. Close your eyes and envision yourself in a calm, quiet setting, such as a beach or forest. Allow yourself to get completely immersed in the sensory aspects of the environment, letting go of any worry or anxiety.

- Gratitude Practice: Think of three things you're grateful for today, no matter how minor or inconsequential they appear. Cultivating a thankfulness mindset may help you change your focus away from stress and negativity and toward positivity and happiness, increasing overall health and relaxation.
- Hydration and Nutrition: Drink lots of water to rehydrate your body after exercise and replace lost fluids. Consume a well-balanced post-workout breakfast or snack that includes carbs, protein, and healthy fats to aid muscle repair and restore energy reserves.

Incorporating these relaxation techniques into your cool-down regimen will help you achieve calm, recuperation, and general well-being after your workout. Experiment with several approaches to see what works best for you, and make relaxing a part of your normal workout routine.

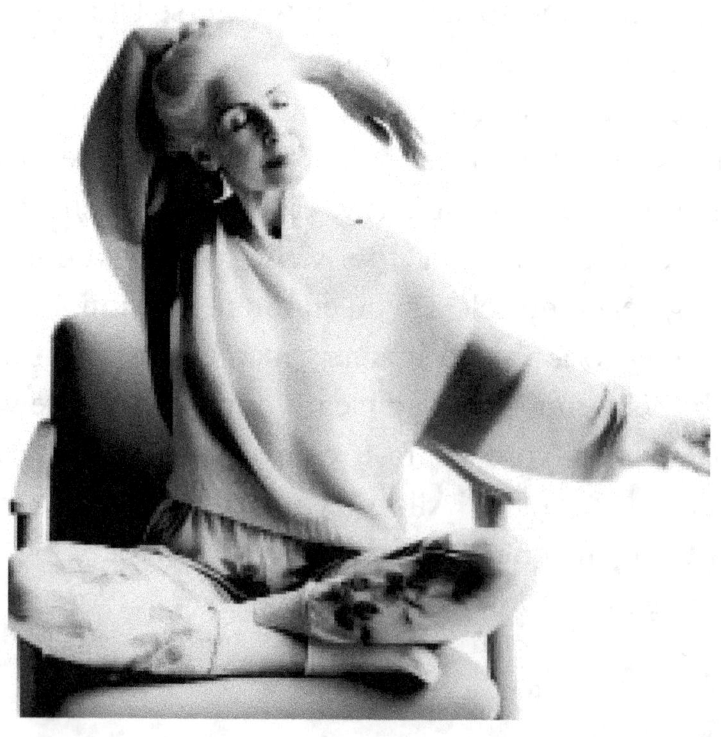

As you progress in
your practice, you'll
develop greater
strength, confidence,
and resilience, both on
and off the mat.
Pilates teaches you
to listen to your
body, trust yourself,
and embrace your
unique journey to
health and vitality.

CHAPTER 4
Progressing with Confidence: Intermediate Routines

Progressing confidently through intermediate exercises entails challenging your body while maintaining appropriate form and technique.

Here's a Guide that will help you advance safely and productively.

- Analyze Your Current Level: Before moving on to intermediate routines, analyze your current fitness level and knowledge with the exercises. Ensure that you have mastered fundamental movements and have developed adequate strength and endurance.
- Set precise, attainable goals for your intermediate exercises, such as building strength, improving flexibility, or learning new abilities. Clear objectives will keep you motivated and focused on your development.
- Gradually raise Intensity: To raise the intensity of your workouts, add resistance, increase repetitions or sets, or incorporate more difficult activities. Aim for slow, sustained improvement to avoid overexertion or damage.
- Pay special attention to your form and technique throughout workouts to guarantee proper muscle engagement and decrease the chance of injury. Throughout each exercise, keep your posture correct, engage your core, and move with control.
- Vary Your Routine: To keep your workouts interesting and difficult, use a range of exercises that target different muscle groups and movement patterns.

Develop a well-rounded fitness regimen by incorporating strength training, aerobic activity, flexibility exercises, and functional movements.

- Push Your Limits: Experiment with new workouts or make established ones more tough. Experiment with various training methods, such as circuit training, interval training, or plyometrics, to push your body in novel ways.

- Listen to Your Body: Pay attention to how your body reacts to exercise and modify your regimen accordingly. If you encounter pain or discomfort, reduce the intensity or adapt the exercises as necessary. Rest and recuperation are critical for success, so schedule enough rest days and recovery procedures.

- Keep note of your exercise, noting any gains in strength, endurance, flexibility, and general performance. Celebrate your triumphs and use them as encouragement to keep moving forward with confidence.

- Seek Professional Help: Consider hiring a professional personal trainer or fitness teacher who can give specific direction, support, and feedback to help you achieve your objectives safely and effectively.

- Maintain Consistency: Consistency is essential for moving confidently. Stick to your training program, prioritize your health and fitness objectives, and believe in your capacity to overcome obstacles and make steady improvement over time.

Following these principles will let you to confidently proceed through intermediate routines, challenging your body while focusing on safety, technique, and general well-being. Remember to listen to your body, maintain consistency, and enjoy your accomplishments along the road.

Wall Plank

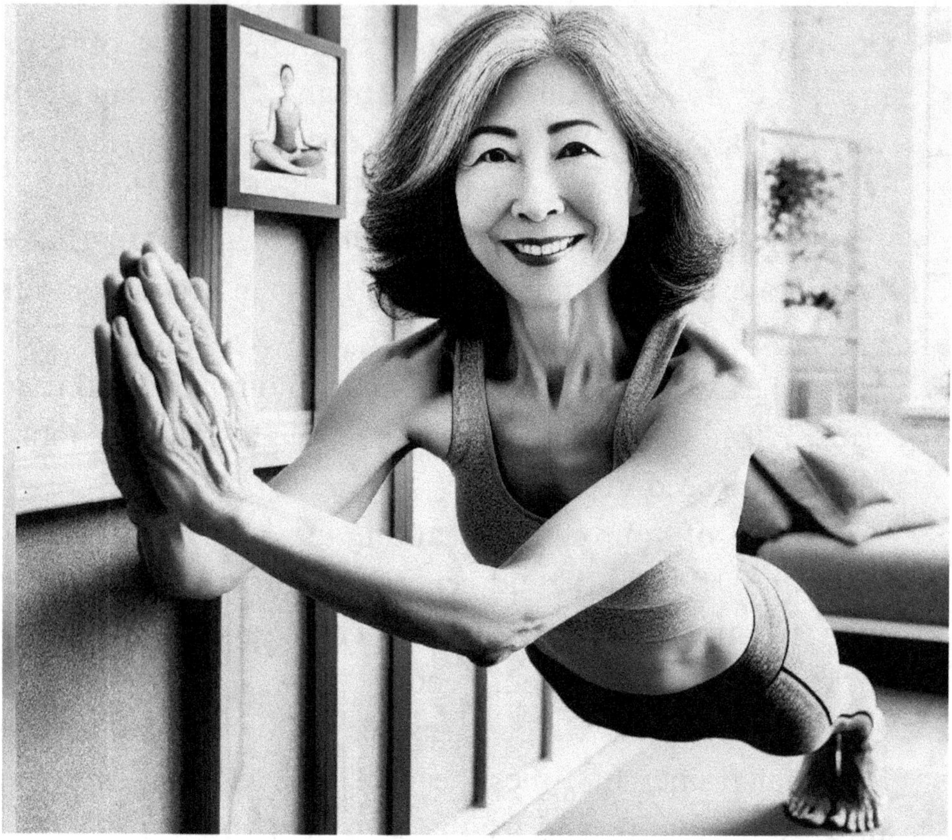

Wall planks are a great variant on the standard plank workout since they test your core and increase upper body strength while offering extra support from the wall.

Here's how to use wall planks effectively:

- Set up: Begin by facing a wall about an arm's length away. Position your hands on the wall at shoulder height, somewhat wider than shoulder width apart. Your arms should be straight, with your fingers pointing up.

- Brace your core muscles by bringing your belly button toward your spine. This involvement will assist to keep your body stable during the workout.
- Step back: Take a few steps away from the wall, keeping your hands firmly planted. Walk your feet back until your body is in a straight line from your head to your heels, arms perpendicular to the floor.
- Adjust Your Position: Keep your feet hip-width apart and your heels exactly beneath your hips. Your shoulders should be placed squarely above your wrists, and your head should be aligned with your spine, facing the wall.
- Maintain the plank posture by maintaining your body firm and preventing drooping or arching in your back. Squeeze your glutes and engage your core to keep your body stable.
- Take calm, deep breaths while maintaining the plank posture. Inhale deeply through your nose and expel completely through your mouth to maintain control and steadiness.
- Hold and Progress: Begin with holding the plank position for 20-30 seconds, then progressively increasing the duration as you gain strength and endurance. For best results, build up to holding the plank for 60 seconds or more.
- Maintain Form: Throughout the workout, focus on your form and technique. Maintain a straight line from head to heels, prevent rising or lowering your hips, and maintain your shoulders steady and engaged.

Modify as Needed: If you find the wall plank too difficult, place your hands on a higher surface, such as a countertop or solid bench, to minimize the angle of your body and the intensity of the exercise.

If you wish to enhance the difficulty, lower your hands to a lower surface, such as a step or low bench.

- Cool Down: After holding the plank for the chosen amount of time, gradually move your feet back toward the wall and come to a standing position. Stretch your arms, shoulders, and core muscles to alleviate stress.

Incorporate wall planks into your normal exercise program to test your core, increase upper body strength, and improve overall stability and posture. With constant practice and advancement, your strength and endurance will increase over time.

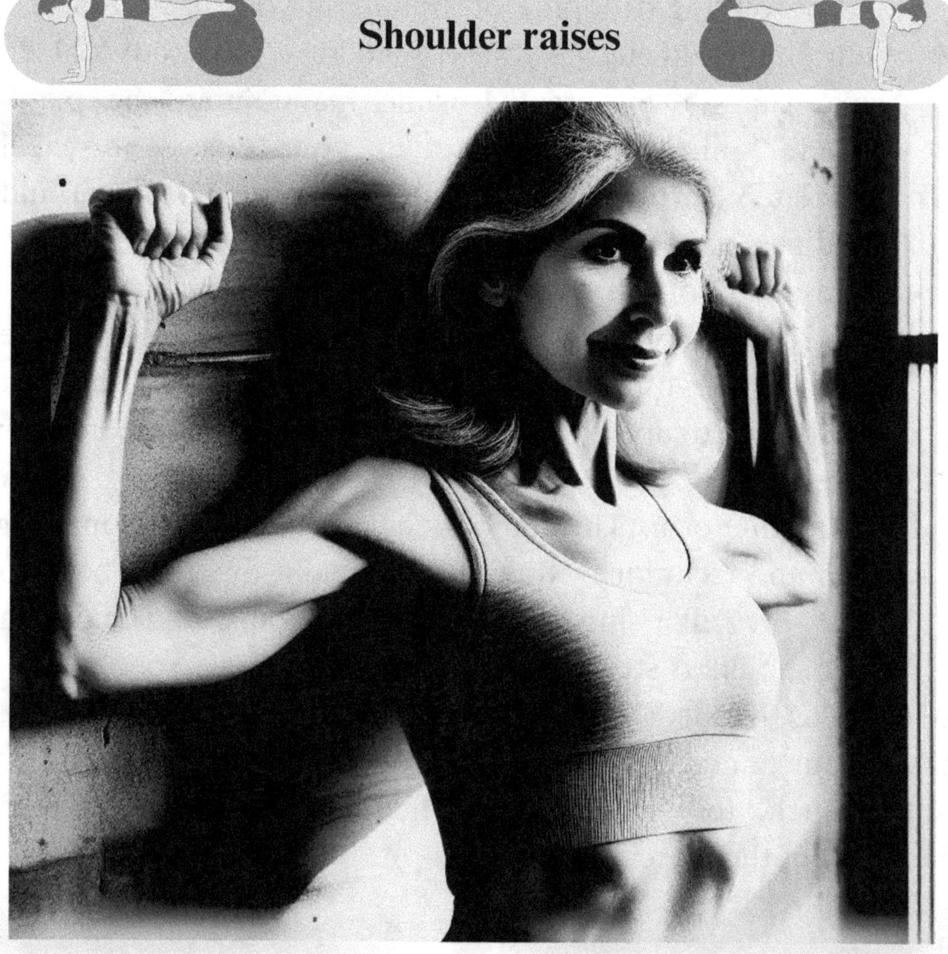

Shoulder raises are a useful workout for increasing shoulder stability and lowering discomfort because they strengthen the muscles surrounding the shoulder joint. Here's how to do shoulder lifts properly.

- Set up: Stand tall, feet hip-width apart, arms relaxed at your sides. Hold a light dumbbell in each hand, palms facing inward to your body.
- Brace your core muscles by bringing your belly button toward your spine. This will help you stabilize your torso and keep appropriate posture during the activity.
- Start position: Keep your elbows slightly bent and your shoulders relaxed. Ensure that your neck is in line with your spine and your sight is ahead.
- Raise Your Arms: Exhale and slowly raise both arms out to the sides, parallel to the floor. Keep your elbows slightly bent during the action, and concentrate on working the muscles around your shoulder blades.
- Control your movement: Don't swing or use momentum to raise the weights. Instead, lift and drop your arms slowly and steadily, focusing on the muscles in your shoulders and upper back.
- Pause at the Top: Once your arms are parallel to the floor, take a moment to press your shoulder blades together and activate the muscles in your upper back. This improves shoulder stability and develops the muscles involved in normal posture.
- drop Your Arms: Inhale and steadily drop your arms back to their starting position, keeping control throughout the exercise. Keep your shoulders relaxed and avoid shrugging them toward your ears.
- Repeat: Perform the shoulder lifts for the appropriate amount of repetitions, beginning with 8-12 reps.

As you gain strength, progressively increase the weight or number of repetitions.

- Maintain proper form and technique throughout the workout. Maintain a slow and controlled motion, and avoid abrupt or rapid motions that might strain your shoulders.
- Modify as needed: If you feel pain or discomfort in your shoulders, reduce the weight of the dumbbells or the range of motion. You may also do the exercise with your arms slightly in front of you rather than straight out to the sides.

Integrating shoulder raises into your normal workout practice will assist improve shoulder stability, reduce soreness, and increase upper body strength. If you have any pre-existing shoulder problems or issues, speak with a fitness professional or physical therapist before doing this exercise

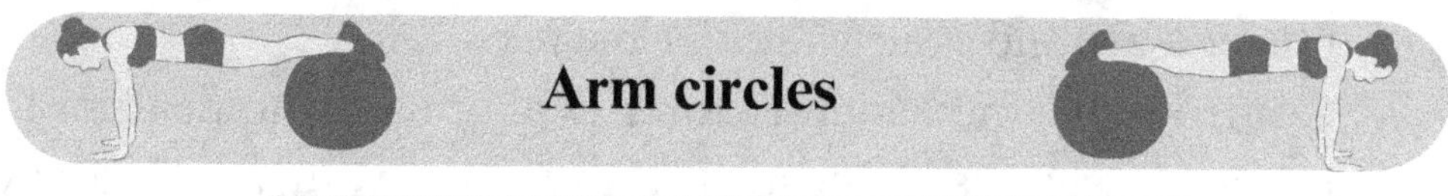

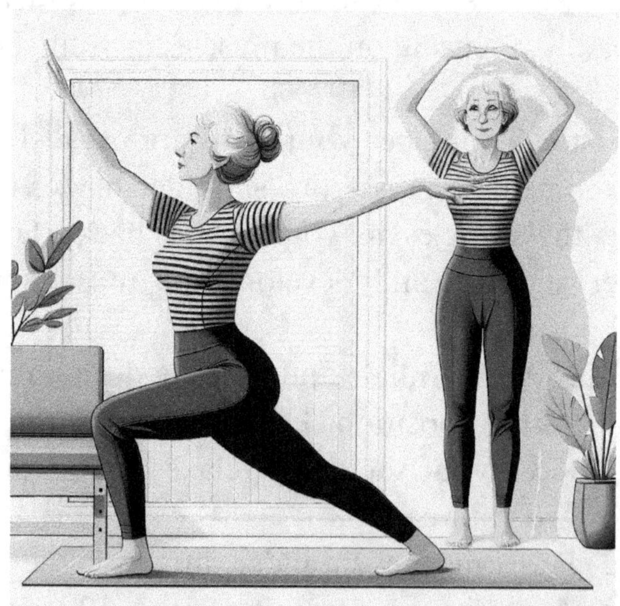

Arm circles are a basic yet effective exercise for improving flexibility and range of motion in the shoulders and arms. Here's how to do arm circles properly

- Set up: Stand tall, feet hip-width apart, arms relaxed at your sides. Make sure your posture is upright, shoulders back, and chest raised.
- Brace your core muscles by bringing your belly button toward your spine. This will help you stabilize your torso and keep appropriate posture during the activity.
- Extend Your Arms: Hold your arms out to the sides at shoulder height, palms facing down towards the floor. To avoid locking out, keep your elbows slightly bent.
- Begin making little circular motions with your arms, pushing them forward in a controlled manner. Imagine tracing circles with your fingertips on the wall in front of you.
- Gradually Increase Size: As you grow more comfortable with the movement, gradually expand the circles, making them larger and broader. Maintain a smooth and flowing motion throughout the workout.
- Concentrate on control: Avoid flailing your arms or utilizing momentum to create circles. Instead, utilize the muscles in your shoulders and arms to regulate the movement and stay stable.
- Adjust the pace of the arm circles according on your preferences and fitness level. Experiment with slow, methodical circles and faster-paced movements to push your muscles in new ways.
- Reverse Direction: After executing forward arm circles for a certain amount of time or repetitions, transition to circular motions in the reverse direction, moving your arms backward.

- This promotes a balanced development of the shoulder muscles.
- Maintain proper alignment throughout the workout by keeping your shoulders relaxed and away from your ears. Keep your chest wide and your spine neutral to avoid straining your neck or upper back.
- Breathe: Keep your breathing steady and regular throughout the activity. Inhale as you circle your arms forward or backward, then exhale as you finish each rotation.

Arm circles should be performed in 1-2 sets of 10-20 repetitions in each direction as part of your warm-up routine or as a standalone exercise to improve shoulder flexibility and range of motion. As your flexibility improves, gradually extend or intensify the circles.

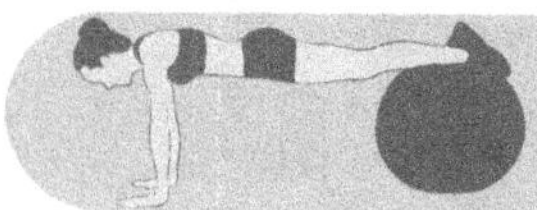

Standing Leg Extension

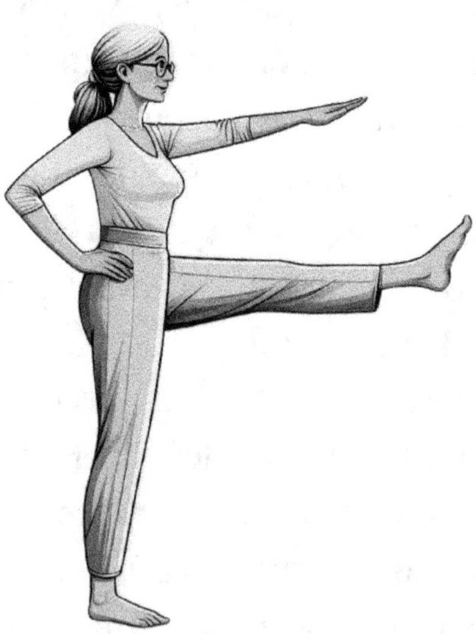

Standing leg extensions are an excellent workout for strengthening the quadriceps and increasing balance and stability. Here's how to do standing leg extensions correctly

- Set up: Stand tall, feet hip-width apart, arms relaxed at your sides. Draw your belly button towards your spine to engage your core muscles and stabilize your torso.
- Find Your Balance: Shift your weight to one leg while maintaining a little bend in the knee. This will be your supporting leg during the activity.
- Lift the Other Leg: Lift your other leg off the ground while maintaining it straight and parallel to the floor. Maintain the elevated leg position by engaging your quadriceps.
- Extend Your Leg: Slowly extend your elevated leg straight out in front of you, trying to reach hip height or slightly higher. Keep your toes pointing forward and your foot flexed to work the leg muscles.
- Pause and Squeeze: Hold the extended position briefly, concentrating on squeezing your quadriceps at the peak of the exercise. This increases muscular activation and strengthens the muscles in your thigh.
- Control the Lowering Phase: Slowly lower your extended leg back to its starting position, keeping control throughout the movement. Keep your movements smooth and purposeful to test your balance and stability.
- Maintain Proper Alignment: Keep your hips level during the workout and prevent leaning or tipping to the side. To avoid excessive effort, maintain an erect torso and relaxed shoulders.
- Repeat on Both Sides: Do the required number of repetitions on one leg before moving to the opposite side. Aim for 8-12 repetitions on each leg to adequately target the quadriceps while also improving balance.

- Modify as needed: If you are having trouble keeping balance, you can use a substantial item like a chair or a countertop for support. As you feel more comfortable with the exercise, progressively reduce the amount of help until you can do it alone.
- Breathe: Keep your breathing steady and regular throughout the activity. Inhale as you lift your leg and exhale as you stretch it, keeping a constant breathing rhythm to help you move.

Include standing leg extensions in your lower body exercise program to target your quadriceps, improve balance, and increase overall lower body strength and stability. As you gain strength and confidence, progressively increase the amount of repetitions or add resistance to further test your muscle.

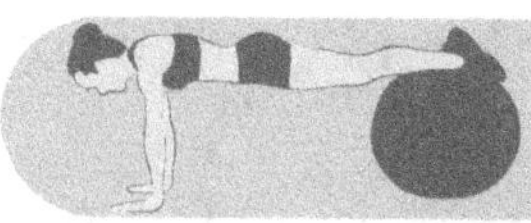 **Wall sit variations** 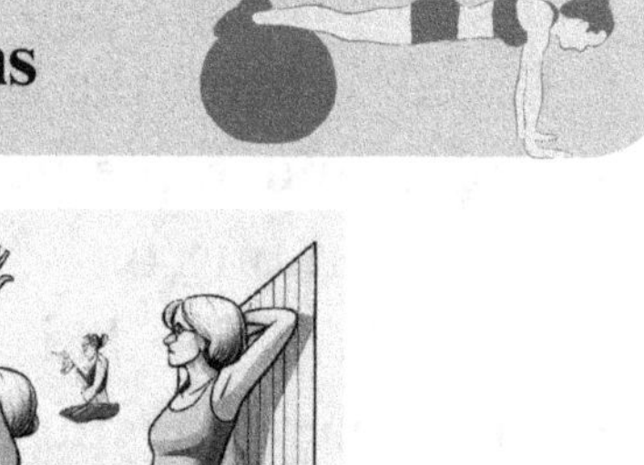

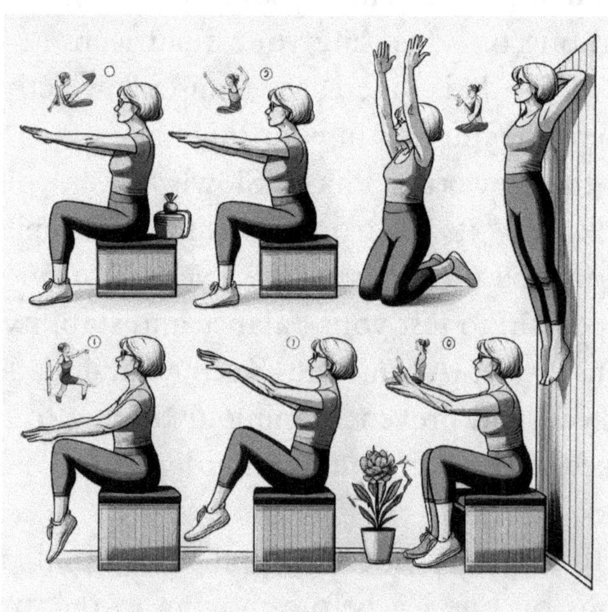

Wall sit variants are great for increasing endurance and strengthening the leg muscles, such as the quadriceps, hamstrings, and gluts. Here are a few variants of the wall sit exercise to work your lower body:

1. **Standard Wall Sit**
   - Begin by leaning against a wall, back flat on the surface and feet shoulder-width apart.
   - Lower your body until your thighs are parallel to the floor, creating a 90-degree angle at the knees.
   - Keep your back flat against the wall and your core active.
   - Hold this posture for as long as you can, ideally 30 seconds to 1 minute or more.
   - Maintain appropriate form and breathe steadily throughout the activity.

2. **One-Legged Wall Sit**
   - Begin in the typical wall sit posture, with your back against the wall and your knees bent at a 90° angle.
   - Lift one foot off the ground and stretch your leg straight ahead of you.
   - Hold this position for as long as you can while keeping your supporting leg firm and your core engaged.
   - Switch legs and repeat on the opposite side to promote even growth of both legs.

3. **Pulse Wall Sit**
   - Begin in the typical wall sit posture, with your back against the wall and your thighs parallel to the floor.
   - Lower your body into a wall sit posture, then pulse up and down a few inches while keeping your legs tensioned.
   - Continue pulsating for 10-15 repetitions, then hold the wall sit posture for another 10-15 seconds before relaxing.

1. **Wall Sit With Leg Lifts:**
   - Begin in the conventional wall sit posture, back against the wall, thighs parallel to the floor.
   - Lift one leg off the ground and stretch it straight ahead of you.
   - Hold this position for a few seconds before lowering your leg back down and repeating on the other side.
   - Continue alternating leg lifts while remaining in the wall sit posture for an extra challenge.

2. **Wall Sit and Arm Raises:**
   - Begin in the typical wall sit posture, with your back against the wall and your thighs parallel to the floor.
   - Hold a light dumbbell in each hand, or use your own weight.
   - Extend your arms straight out in front of you, shoulder height and parallel to the floor.
   - Hold this posture while maintaining the wall sit for as long as possible using your shoulders and upper back muscles.

Include these wall sit variants into your lower-body exercise program to increase endurance, leg strength, and diversity. Begin with 2-3 sets of each variation, changing the time or intensity as necessary to match your fitness level.

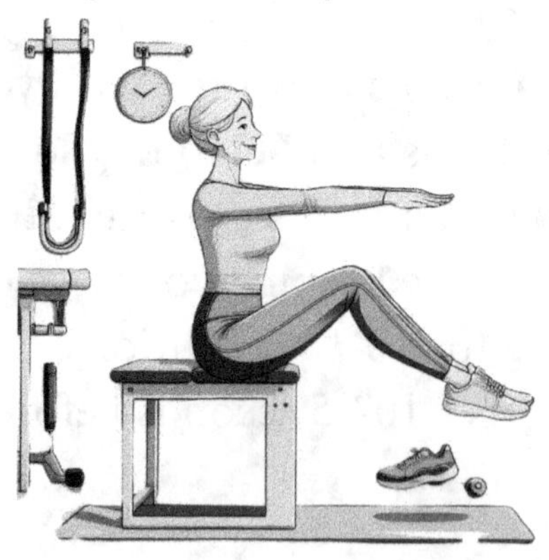

"Keep the momentum going with Wall Pilates: Each day is a new opportunity to thrive."

CHAPTER 5

Finding Your Flow: Advanced Routines

Advanced routines are all about finding your flow—a smooth series of movements that test your body and mind while increasing strength, flexibility, and mindfulness.

Here's how to develop an advanced regimen that will help you discover your flow:

- Begin with a powerful warm-up to get your body ready for the forthcoming challenges. Incorporate exercises that move your joints, stimulate your muscles, and raise your heart rate. Leg swings, arm circles, twisting lunges, and high knees are examples of exercises that might be included.

- Strength Training Circuit: Create a circuit using complex workouts to target various muscle groups. Include difficult exercises like squats, lunges, push-ups, rows, and deadlifts. Perform each exercise with perfect form and control, emphasizing quality over quantity. Aim for 3-4 sets of 8-12 repetitions for each exercise, with little pause between sets to keep your heart rate up.

- Plyometric Drills: Use intense plyometric workouts to increase power and agility. Incorporate exercises such as jump squats, box jumps, burpees, and plyometric push-ups. Perform each exercise with maximal intensity for a predetermined number of repetitions, with an emphasis on explosive movements and fast transitions between exercises.

- Balance and stability. Work on your balance and stability by doing workouts that target your core and proprioceptive muscles.

Include exercises like single-leg deadlifts, stability ball workouts, and balancing board drills. Maintain control and stability throughout each movement by using your core and stabilizing muscles to avoid wobbling or falling.

- Flexibility and Mobility: Make time to develop your flexibility and mobility, which are essential for avoiding injuries and maximizing performance. Incorporate dynamic stretches, yoga postures, and foam rolling to relieve tension, improve range of motion, and speed up muscle recovery. Deep breathing and mindful movement can help you connect with your body and relax.
- Interval Training: Use high-intensity interval training (HIIT) to improve cardiovascular fitness and burn calories. Alternate periods of intensive activity with active recuperation, such as sprint intervals followed by walking or cycling. Adjust the intensity and duration of the intervals to match your fitness level and objectives.
- Mindfulness and Meditation: Finish your advanced regimen with mindfulness and meditation to improve mental clarity and relaxation. Spend a few minutes practicing deep breathing, body scans, or guided meditation to calm your mind and create inner peace. Concentrate on being in the present moment and enjoying the feelings in your body.
- Finish with a thorough cool-down and stretching regimen to decrease muscular pain and enhance healing. Perform static stretches for key muscle groups, concentrating on regions that feel tight or tense. Hold each stretch for 20-30 seconds while breathing deeply to promote relaxation and release.

By incorporating these aspects into your advanced regimen, you may discover your flow and get the deep advantages of a hard yet gratifying workout. Customize your regimen to meet your tastes and fitness objectives, and remember to listen to your body and make changes as required. Enjoy the path of self-discovery and constant progress as you push your boundaries and realize your full potential.

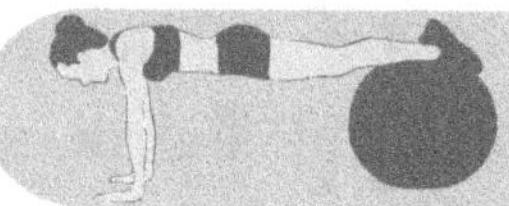 **Pilates Push Ups** 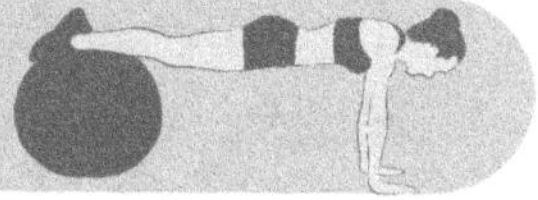

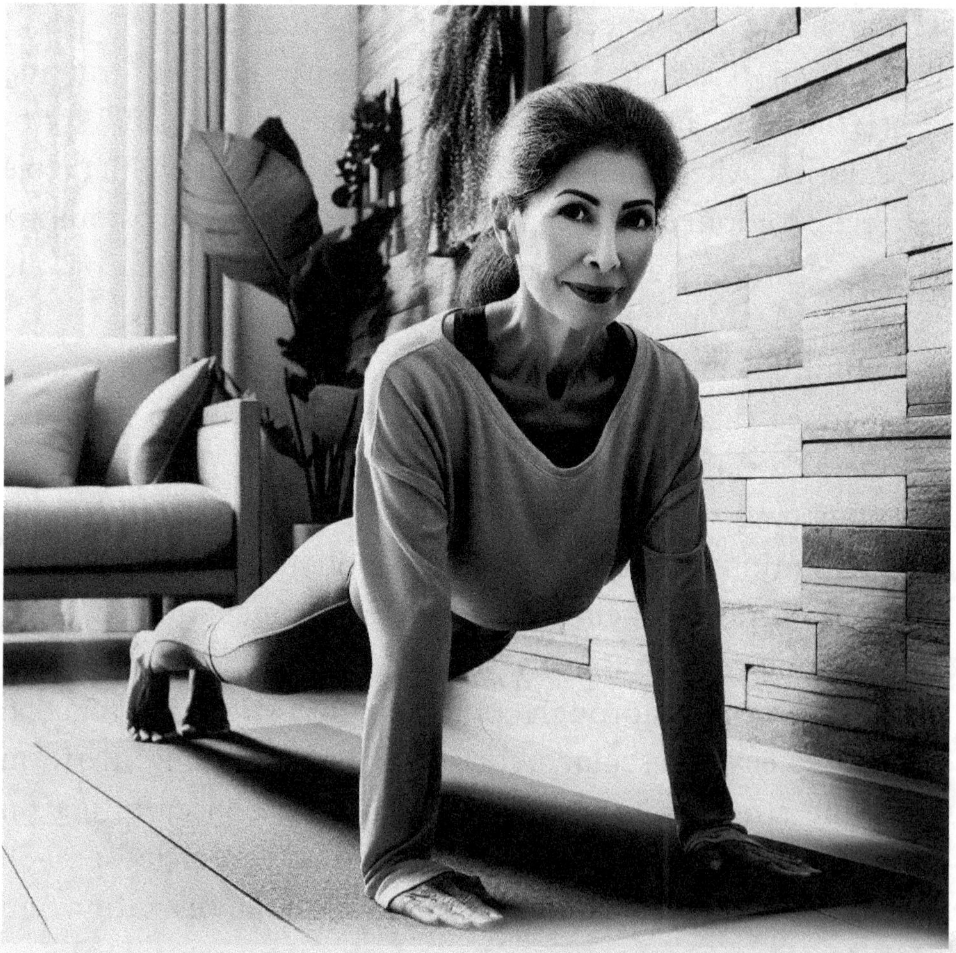

Pilates push-ups are an excellent exercise for developing the upper body, core, and stabilizer muscles while also encouraging good posture and control. Here's how to tweak Pilates push-ups for different levels while maximizing their benefits:

1. **Basic Pilates Push-Up (For Beginners)**
   - Begin in a kneeling position, with your hands just under your shoulders and your legs hip width apart.
   - Engage your core muscles by bringing your belly button towards your spine and keeping your legs and head in a straight line.
   - Lower your chest to the floor by bending your elbows and keeping them close to your body.
   - Push yourself back up to the beginning position, keeping your core stable and avoiding drooping or arching in your back.
   - Perform 8-12 repetitions of controlled motions, paying attention to appropriate form and alignment throughout.

2. **Full Pilates Push-Ups (Intermediate/Advanced)**
   - Begin in a plank stance, hands exactly beneath shoulders and body straight from head to heels.
   - Maintain overall body stability by engaging your core and glutes.
   - Bend your elbows close to your ribs and maintain a straight line from head to heels as you lower your chest to the floor.
   - Push yourself back up to the starting position, focusing on controlled movements and core stability.
   - Perform 8-12 reps with perfect technique, progressively increasing the difficulty as you gain strength.

3. Modified Pilates push-up (intermediate)

- Begin in a plank posture, with your hands on a raised surface like a step, bench, or solid chair.
- Maintain a straight line from head to heels, using your core and glutes for stability.
- Bend your elbows to lower your chest towards the raised surface while remaining in perfect alignment throughout the exercise.
- Push yourself back up to the starting position, focusing on controlled movements and core stability.
- Perform 8-12 repetitions with perfect technique, altering the surface height as needed to challenge yourself.

4. Advanced Pilates Push-Up with a Single Leg

- Begin in a plank stance, hands exactly beneath shoulders and body straight from head to heels.
- Lift one foot off the ground and stretch your leg straight behind you, using your core and glutes for support.
- Bend your elbows to lower your chest to the floor while keeping them tight to your body and maintaining stability through your core and supporting leg.
- Push yourself back up to the starting position, focusing on controlled movements and core stability.
- Perform 8-12 reps on each leg, switching sides between each repeat.

3. Slow-motion Pilates Push-Up (All Levels)

- Perform a conventional Pilates push-up while slowing down the descending component of the exercise.
- Lower your chest slowly and steadily to the floor, counting to 3 or 4 as you descend.
- Pause momentarily at the bottom of the movement, then return to the starting position at a steady speed.

- Maintain stability and perfect form throughout the exercise, and use your core and stabilizer muscles to regulate the movement.

Adapting Pilates push-ups for different levels and focusing on appropriate technique and control, you may optimize their advantages while progressively progressing to more difficult varieties. Remember to listen to your body, begin at the proper level for your fitness level, and progressively raise the challenge as you gain strength and confidence

Single Leg-Kick

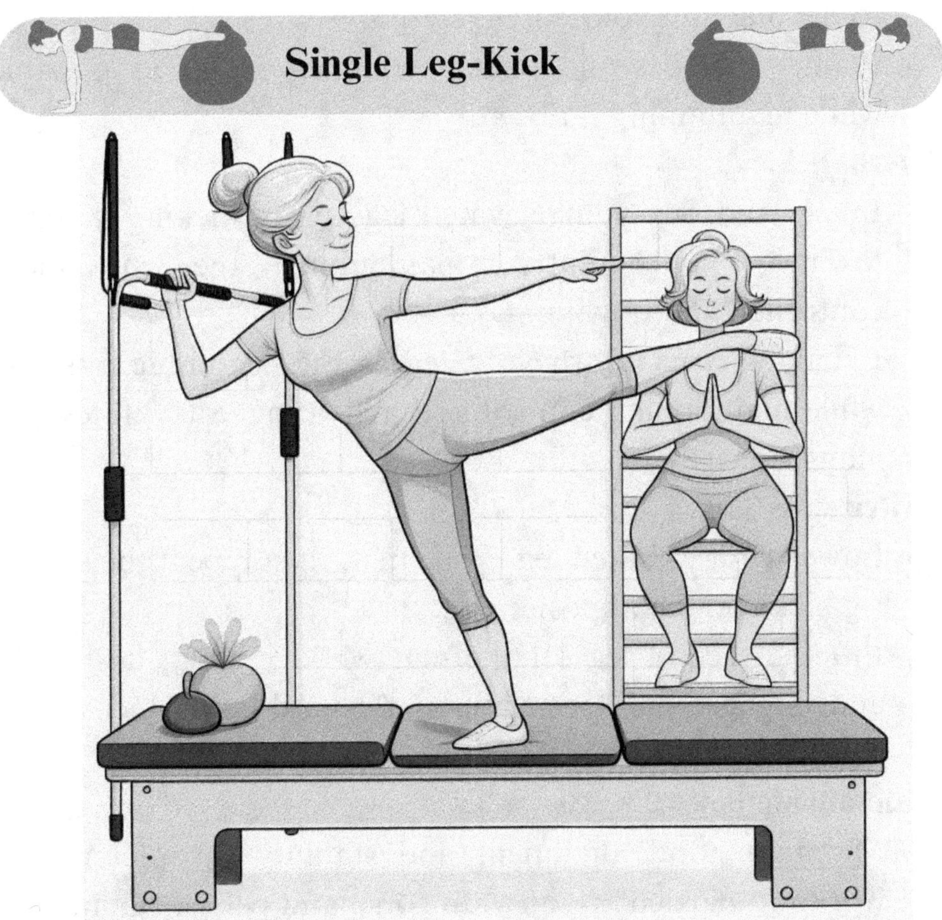

Single-leg kicks are a Pilates exercise that helps to improve balance, coordination, and core strength. Here's how to do single-leg kicks effectively

Starting Position

- Begin by reclining face down on a mat, knees straight and arms folded under your forehead for support. During the exercise, keep your forehead resting on your hands.
- Draw your belly button closer to your spine and stretch your spine to activate your core muscles.

Single-leg Lift

- Lift one leg off the mat by a few inches while maintaining it straight and engaged. Make sure your hips are attached to the mat and your core is stable.
- Point your toes and stretch your leg as far as possible while maintaining it raised.

Alternate kicks

- Inhale and flex your elevated leg before kicking it thrice towards your glutes, maintaining the movement controlled and flowing.
- Exhale as you return your leg to the beginning position while maintaining control and activating your glutes and hamstrings.

Switch sides

- Lower your elevated leg to the mat, then repeat the single-leg kicks on the opposite side.
- Lift the second leg off the mat while keeping it straight and engaged, and repeat the flex-and-point kicks with control and accuracy.

Maintain alignment

- Maintain good alignment and stability throughout the workout, particularly in your torso and pelvis. Maintain a comfortable posture with your shoulders away from your ears. Avoid arching or rounding your lower back.

- Engage your core muscles to support your spine and pelvis, ensuring that the movement comes from your hips and legs, not your lower back.

Breathe mindfully.

- Coordinate your breathing with the movement, inhaling as you flex and kick your leg towards your glutes and exhaling as you stretch your leg back to the beginning position.
- Maintain a consistent and regular breathing pattern throughout the workout to enhance calm and concentration.

Controlled movement

- Concentrate on doing single-leg kicks with control and accuracy, avoiding jerky or abrupt movements. With each kick, focus on stretching and strengthening your leg muscles while keeping your body aligned and stable.

Repetitions

- Aim for 8-10 repetitions of single-leg kicks on each side, concentrating on quality over number. Gradually increase the amount of repetitions as you gain strength and comfort with the exercise.

Incorporate single-leg kicks into your Pilates program to improve your legs' balance, coordination, and core strength. To get the most out of the exercise and develop general body awareness, practice it with control, accuracy, and focus

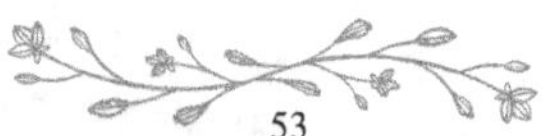

"With Wall Pilates, motivation is built into every movement: Feel the burn, revel in the progress."

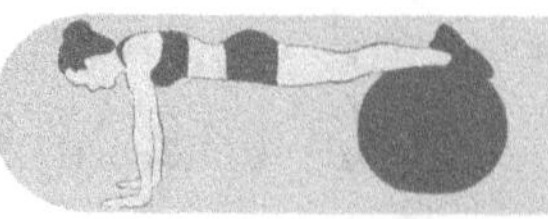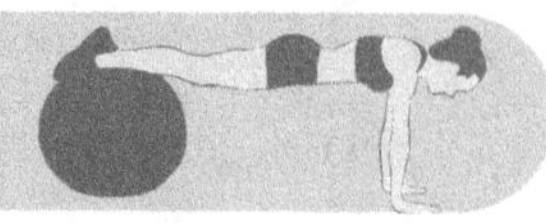

Wall Burpees

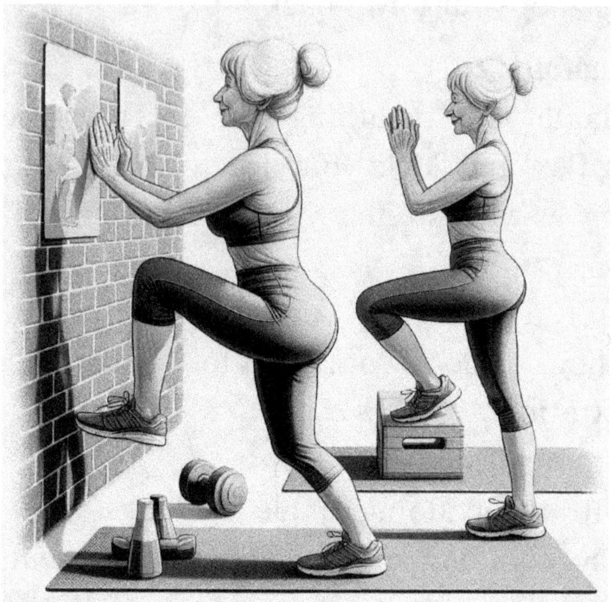

Wall burpees are a dynamic exercise that mixes Pilates and cardio to create a total-body workout. Here's how to do wall burpees successfully.

Starting Position

- Stand facing a solid wall, feet hip-width apart, arms by your sides.
- Draw your belly button towards your spine to engage your core muscles, and keep your shoulders relaxed while you stand tall.
- Squat with hands to the wall:
- Bend your knees and drop your hips back and down to achieve a squat stance.
- Place your hands flat on the wall in front of you, shoulder-width apart, with your wrists immediately beneath your shoulders.

Jump back to plank

- Jump both feet back into a plank stance while maintaining your body straight from head to heels. Engage your core while stabilizing your shoulders and wrists.

Optional push-ups

- If desired, do a push-up by bending your elbows and lowering your chest to the wall. Keep your elbows tight to your torso and your body straight during the exercise.

Jump forward and stand.

- Jump both feet forward toward the wall, landing lightly with both feet flat on the ground.
- Use the strength of your legs to drive yourself higher, raising your arms aloft as you jump.
- Land on soft knees and return to a standing posture, ready to start the next exercise.

Repeat

- Continue the series of actions, flowing easily from one step to the next.
- Throughout the workout, try to keep a consistent speed and focus on appropriate form and alignment.

Breathing

- Coordinate your breath with the motions, inhaling as you descend into the squat and place your hands on the wall, and exhaling as you return to plank or push-up.
- Continue to breathe evenly and rhythmically throughout the workout to support your movements and keep your energy levels up.

Modification:

- If leaping back into plank is too difficult, walk back one foot at a time instead of jumping.

- You may also skip the push-ups if necessary, or do it with your knees on the ground for more assistance.

Repetitions

- Depending on your fitness level and goals, aim for 8-12 wall burpee repeats or a predetermined length of 30 seconds to 1 minute.

By introducing wall burpees into your Pilates exercise, you can add an aerobic component while still concentrating on core engagement, stability, and overall strength. Begin with a moderate number of repetitions and progressively increase as you gain familiarity with the exercise. Remember to listen to your body and make adjustments as needed to maintain safety and appropriate technique.

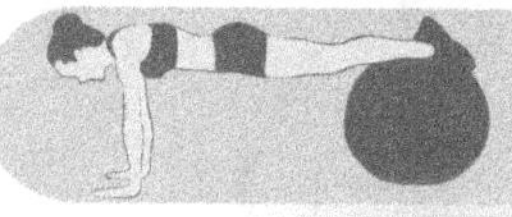

Spine stretches.

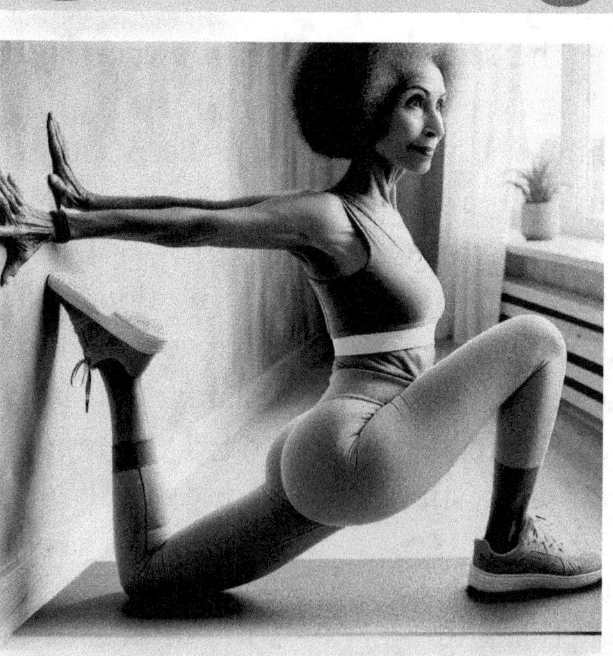

Spine stretches are vital for maintaining flexibility, enhancing posture, and relieving back discomfort. Here are some helpful spine stretches to include in your routine:

Cat-Cow Stretch

- Begin on your hands and knees, placing your wrists precisely under your shoulders and your knees beneath your hips.
- Inhale as you arch your back, bringing your belly to the ground and raising your chest and tailbone to the ceiling (Cow Pose).
- Exhale while rounding your back, tucking your chin into your chest and bringing your belly button toward your spine (Cat Pose).
- For 8-10 repetitions, move smoothly between the Cat and Cow positions while breathing.

Child's Pose

- Begin on your hands and knees, then sit back on your heels, keeping your knees wide apart.
- Walk your hands forward, then drop your chest to the mat, resting your forehead on the ground.
- Stretch your back and shoulders by reaching your arms forward or sideways.
- Hold the stretch for 30 seconds to one minute, concentrating on deep breathing and relaxation.

Seated Forward Fold

- Sit on the floor, legs straight in front of you, feet flexed.
- Inhale as you stretch your spine, then exhale as you bend forward at the hips and reach for your feet.
- Hold onto your shins, ankles, or feet, depending on your flexibility, and slowly draw yourself closer to your legs.
- Maintain a long spine and prevent rounding the back.

Hold the stretch for 30 seconds to a minute, inhaling deeply into it.

Twisting the Supine Spinal Twist
- Lie on your back, arms stretched to the sides in a T posture, knees bent.
- Exhale as you lower both knees to one side, keeping your shoulders firmly planted on the mat.
- Gently twist your body to look in the opposite direction of your knees, experiencing a stretch in your spine and chest.
- Hold the stretch for 30 seconds to a minute before returning to the middle and repeating on the opposite side.

Standing Forward Fold
- Stand with your feet hip-width apart, knees slightly bent.
- Inhale as you raise your arms overhead, then exhale as you bend forward at the hips and reach for the floor.
- Allow your head and neck to relax as your arms dangle lightly to the ground.
- Hold the stretch for 30 seconds to 1 minute, focusing on stretching your spine and hamstrings.

Sphinx Pose
- Lie on your stomach, elbows bent and forearms flat on the mat, beneath your shoulders.
- Press into your forearms and raise your chest off the mat, stretching your spine and expanding your chest.
- Keep your shoulders relaxed and away from your ears, and use your core to support your lower back.
- Hold the stretch for 30 seconds to a minute while inhaling deeply into your abdomen and chest.
- Add these spine exercises to your daily routine to increase flexibility, relieve tension, and enhance overall spinal health.

Remember to listen to your body and refrain from pushing any motions that produce pain or discomfort. If you have any current back ailments or injuries, speak with a doctor before beginning a new stretching regimen.

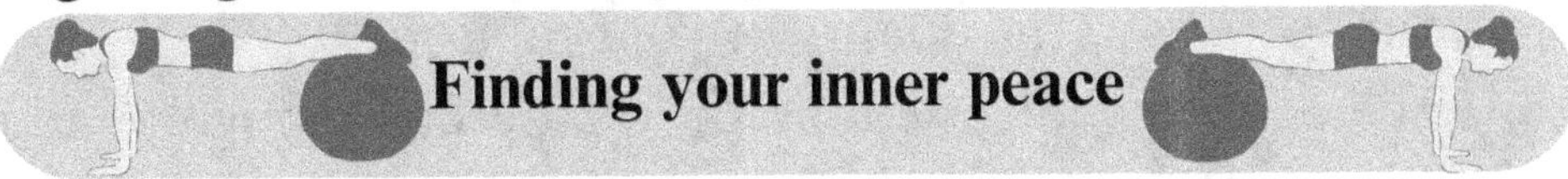

Finding your inner peace

Meditation and mindfulness activities can help you relax, focus, and become more aware of your body, enhancing your Pilates experience. Here are some meditation and mindfulness practices you may use in your Pilates practice:

Mindful breathing:

- Begin your Pilates practice with a few minutes of focused breathing to help you center yourself and relax.
- Find a comfortable seated or sleeping posture, close your eyes, and focus on your breath.
- Take slow, deep breaths in through your nose and expel completely through your mouth, concentrating on the sensation of your breath entering and exiting your body.
- Notice how your abdomen rises and falls with each breath, then exhale to release any stress or distractions.

Body Scan Meditation:

- After warming up your body, do a body scan meditation to increase awareness of physical sensations.
- Close your eyes and focus your attention on different areas of your body, beginning with your head and continuing down to your toes.
- Identify any points of tension or discomfort and intentionally relax those muscles with each exhale.
- As you practice Pilates movements, be conscious of your spine's alignment, core muscle activation, and limb lengthening.

Focused Attention

- During Pilates moves, focus your attention on your body's feelings and motions.
- Concentrate on the muscles you're using, the position of your spine, and the quality of your motions.
- Let go of any distractions or wandering thoughts, and with each breath, return your focus to the present moment.

Visualization

- Use visualization methods to improve your Pilates practice by picturing yourself moving with ease and elegance.
- Imagine yourself completing each exercise with perfect form and control, feeling the muscles contract and extend with each movement.
- Visualize the benefits of your Pilates practice, such as greater strength, flexibility, and energy.

Gratitude Practice

- During your Pilates exercise, think on the various advantages it provides to your body and mind.
- Take a minute to be thankful for your body's strength, resiliency, and capacity to move.
- Appreciate the chance to take time for yourself and nurture your body via activity and mindfulness.

Closing Meditation

- Finish your Pilates session with a closing meditation to fully integrate the physical and mental benefits of your practice.
- Sit or lie down in a comfortable posture, close your eyes, and take some time to think on your experience.

- Express thanks for your body and mind, and make a commitment to carry the tranquility and awareness you gained during your practice throughout the remainder of your day.

Incorporate these meditation and mindfulness activities into your Pilates program to improve your general well-being and strengthen your relationship with your body and breath. Experiment with different ways to see what resonates best with you, and enjoy the journey of self-discovery and inner calm via movement.

"Keep the momentum going with Wall Pilates: Each day is a new opportunity to thrive."

CHAPTER 6

Your Personalized Pilates Journey

Your Pilates journey is a revolutionary route designed individually for your requirements, goals, and unique body. It is a comprehensive approach to fitness and well-being that includes not just physical activity, but also mindfulness, self-awareness, and general health improvement.

At first, we do an in-depth evaluation to determine your current fitness level, any existing health concerns, and your unique Pilates goals. Whether you want to improve your flexibility, gain strength, relieve pain, or foster a stronger mind-body connection, this examination will help you create a personalized program that will help you achieve your objectives.

Your personalized Pilates experience begins with a carefully crafted sequence of exercises that grow and adapt to your progress. Each session is thoughtfully planned to both challenge and assist you, using a variety of mat exercises, equipment-based routines, and specialty movements customized to your body's specific requirements.

Mindfulness activities are crucial to your journey because they increase your mind-body connection and improve the whole experience. Through concentrated breathing, body awareness exercises, and visualization methods, you will learn to coordinate your movements with your breath, increase your awareness of physiological sensations, and build a profound sense of present and peace.

Beyond the physical components, your individualized Pilates journey takes a comprehensive approach to wellbeing that includes nutrition, hydration, and lifestyle behaviors.

By addressing these essential aspects of well-being, we provide a holistic framework for optimal health and vitality that supplements your Pilates practice and improves your entire quality of life.

Throughout your journey, you will receive continual support, direction, and encouragement to keep you motivated and inspired. Regular progress reviews guarantee that your program is dynamic and successful, while a supportive community creates a loving atmosphere in which you may grow and celebrate your accomplishments.

Your Pilates journey is a revolutionary journey of self-discovery, empowerment, and overall wellbeing. It's a path that recognizes your uniqueness, celebrates your accomplishments, and enables you to reach your maximum potential for health, happiness, and vitality.

Creating your own workout plan

Creating your own exercise plan allows you to customize your fitness program to your own objectives, tastes, and fitness level. Here's how you may create a personalized training plan by choosing exercises and modifying intensity:

Set your goals.

- Begin by outlining your exercise goals, whether they be to gain strength, improve cardiovascular health, increase flexibility, or lose weight. Clear objectives will help influence your workout choices and intensity.

Choose your exercises.

- Choose workouts that target various muscle groups and areas of fitness. Squats, lunges, push-ups, and rows are examples of strength training activities that can help in muscular growth. Incorporate cardiovascular workouts like jogging, cycling, or jumping jacks to improve heart health and burn calories. Flexibility activities, such as yoga postures or Pilates stretches, can help increase mobility and avoid injuries.

Consider your preferences.

- Choose workouts you enjoy and are likely to keep to. If you despise jogging, try cycling or swimming instead. Experiment with various sorts of exercises, such as HIIT, circuit training, or dance-based workouts, to see what motivates and engages you.

Assess your fitness level.

- Be open and honest about your current fitness level, as well as any limits or ailments. Begin with exercises that are appropriate for your ability, then improve as you gain strength and confidence. If you're unsure, ask a fitness professional for advice.

Tailor Intensity

- Adjust the intensity of your workouts based on your objectives and fitness level. Increase the weight, resistance, or duration of your workouts to push your muscles and cardiovascular system. Interval training, which alternates between high-intensity bursts and times of rest or reduced intensity, can help you burn more calories and increase your fitness efficiency.

Create a balanced routine.

- Create a comprehensive fitness schedule that incorporates strength training, aerobic activity, flexibility work, and recuperation days. To attain complete results, use a variety of workouts that target different sections of the body and components of fitness.

Progress Gradually

- Gradually increase the intensity, duration, or complexity of your exercises over time to maintain growth and prevent plateaus. Listen to your body and modify your strategy as required to avoid overtraining or burnout.

Track your progress.

- Keep a workout diary or use a fitness monitoring app to log your exercises, monitor your progress, and celebrate your accomplishments. Monitoring your performance may help you stay motivated while also identifying opportunities for improvement.

Listen to your body.

- Pay attention to how your body reacts to exercise and modify your strategy accordingly. Rest and recuperate as required, and avoid pushing yourself above your limitations. Consistency and sustainability are critical for long-term success.

You may develop a tailored workout regimen that is successful, pleasurable, and sustainable by carefully picking activities and adjusting the intensity to your objectives and fitness level. As you continue on your fitness path, remember to remain flexible and adaptable, as well as open to new experiences.

Listening to your Body

Listening to your body is essential for identifying and avoiding pain when exercising. Here are some recommendations to help you listen to your body's messages and avoid injury:

1. Know the difference. Between discomfort and pain Discomfort during exercise, such as muscular tiredness or minor soreness, is natural and generally indicative of your muscles working. However, strong or intense pain is abnormal and may suggest an injury. Learn to distinguish between the two feelings and discontinue exercise if you feel discomfort.
2. Start Slowly and Progress Gradually Introduce new workouts or workout routines gradually, especially if you are a novice or returning to exercise after a break. Listen to your body and gradually increase the intensity, duration, or complexity of your exercises to avoid overexertion and injury.
3. Focus on technique and form. To avoid strain and injury, exercise should be performed with good technique and form. Poor form can place unneeded strain on your joints and muscles, increasing the likelihood of pain and damage. If you are unclear about appropriate form, see a professional personal trainer or fitness instructor.
4. Warm up and cool down properly. Always begin your exercises with a full warm-up to get your body ready for activity and enhance blood flow to your muscles. Similarly, after your workout, cool down with mild stretching or foam rolling to enhance muscle healing and minimize pain

Listening to your body is essential for identifying and avoiding pain when exercising. Here are some recommendations to help you listen to your body's messages and avoid injury:

1. Know the difference. Between discomfort and pain Discomfort during exercise, such as muscular tiredness or minor soreness, is natural and generally indicative of your muscles working. However, strong or intense pain is abnormal and may suggest an injury. Learn to distinguish between the two feelings and discontinue exercise if you feel discomfort.
2. Start Slowly and Progress Gradually Introduce new workouts or workout routines gradually, especially if you are a novice or returning to exercise after a break. Listen to your body and gradually increase the intensity, duration, or complexity of your exercises to avoid overexertion and injury.
3. Focus on technique and form. To avoid strain and injury, exercise should be performed with good technique and form. Poor form can place unneeded strain on your joints and muscles, increasing the likelihood of pain and damage. If you are unclear about appropriate form, see a professional personal trainer or fitness instructor.
4. Warm up and cool down properly. Always begin your exercises with a full warm-up to get your body ready for activity and enhance blood flow to your muscles. Similarly, after your workout, cool down with mild stretching or foam rolling to enhance muscle healing and minimize pain

5. Listen to Joint and Muscle Feedback.

Pay alert to any signs of pain or tension in your joints and muscles when exercising. If you detect any strange sensations in your joints, such as clicking, popping, or grinding, or if you have chronic tightness or discomfort in a specific muscle area, take a break and evaluate the issue.

6. alter or Avoid Painful motions

If specific workouts or motions cause pain or discomfort, alter or avoid them completely. There are frequently alternate workouts or modifications that target the same muscle areas without causing discomfort or damage.

7. Rest and recover.

Listen to your body's need for rest and healing. Allow enough time between exercises for your muscles to heal and regenerate, and emphasize good sleep and diet to help your body recover.

8. Seek professional guidance.

If you are experiencing chronic or severe discomfort when exercising, speak with a healthcare expert, such as a physical therapist or sports medicine specialist. They can evaluate your health, offer advice on pain management, and suggest suitable exercises or treatments to address any underlying difficulties.

Remember, paying attention to your body's signals, using good exercise technique, and prioritizing rest and recovery, you may avoid discomfort and injury while exercising and get the numerous advantages of a safe and successful workout regimen. Remember that your body's well-being should always be your main concern, so pay attention to its signs and adapt your strategy appropriately.

Staying Motivated

Staying motivated is critical for sticking to a steady training plan and reaching your fitness objectives. Setting objectives, evaluating progress, and celebrating accomplishment can help you stay motivated.

1. Setting Goals.

Define specific, attainable goals that will inspire and challenge you. Whether it's running a 5K, reducing weight, building strength, or improving flexibility, having defined objectives gives you something to strive for and keeps you focused and motivated.

2. Setting SMART Goals

Make your goals SMART (specific, measurable, attainable, relevant, and time-bound). For example, instead of saying "I want to get in shape," make a goal like "I want to lose 10 pounds in three months by exercising three times per week and eating a balanced diet."

3. Breaking Goals Down

Divide big goals into smaller, attainable activities or milestones. This makes your objectives feel more reachable and helps you measure your progress more efficiently. Celebrate each milestone along the road to keep your motivation up.

4. Tracking progress

Track your progress using a workout journal, fitness app, or spreadsheet. Record your exercises, measurements, and successes on a regular basis to evaluate how far you've gone and where you may improve.

5. Measurement of Success

Use both quantitative and subjective criteria to track your success. Weight, body measurements, and workout performance are examples of objective indicators, whereas subjective measures include your mood, energy levels, and overall well-being.

6. Celebrate achievement, no matter how tiny.

Whether you've reached a milestone, set a personal best, or stuck to your fitness routine for a month straight, take the time to recognize and thank yourself for your efforts and devotion.

7. Find Accountability Partners

Share your objectives with friends, family, or a workout partner who can provide encouragement, motivation, and accountability. Having someone to share your accomplishments and struggles with might help you stay motivated and accountable.

8. Visualize Your Success.

Visualize yourself attaining your objectives and how you will feel when you do. Use visualization methods to mentally practice your routines and see yourself overcoming hurdles and succeeding.

9. Adaptation and Adjusting

Be adaptable and open to change your goals and techniques as necessary. If you run into failures or barriers, don't be discouraged—use them as learning opportunities and change your strategy accordingly.

10. Rewarding yourself

Treat yourself to rewards or incentives as you hit milestones or achieve your goals.

Rewards, such as a new exercise attire, a massage, or a relaxing day off, may help reinforce positive behaviors and keep you motivated to stick to your goals.

Setting goals, measuring progress, and celebrating achievement will help you stay motivated and focused on attaining your fitness objectives. Remember to be patient, consistent, and devoted to your goals, and you will be on your path to success.

Building a supportive community

Building a supportive group of like-minded women may be extremely inspiring and encouraging during your fitness journey. Here's how to meet other women who have similar fitness objectives and values:

1. Join fitness classes or groups.

Participate in exercise courses or clubs designed exclusively for women. Whether you enjoy yoga, Pilates, jogging, or strength training, finding a group of women who share your hobbies may give a feeling of community and support.

2. Attend women's workshops or events.

Look for classes, seminars, or activities geared at women's fitness and wellbeing. These events frequently offer opportunity to interact with other women, hear from professionals, and share personal experiences in a friendly setting.

3. Join online communities.

Investigate online forums, social media groups, and fitness applications geared for women's fitness and wellness. These virtual communities provide a forum for women all around the world to interact, share ideas and advice, and celebrate their accomplishments together.

4. Participate in challenge or accountability groups.

Join fitness challenges or accountability groups made particularly for women. These organizations frequently offer a structured framework, daily check-ins, and support from other members to keep you motivated and responsible.

5. Go to women's retreats or retreat centers.

Consider attending a women's fitness retreat or visiting a retreat place with women-specific programming. These retreats provide an immersive experience that allows you to interact with other women, participate in physical activities, and revitalize your mind, body, and soul.

6. Plan meetups or group workouts.

Take the initiative and organize meetups or group exercises with other women in your town. Whether it's a weekend stroll, a morning yoga session in the park, or a group fitness class at the gym, scheduling social meetings may help you make lasting connections and friendships.

7. Seek out female fitness professionals.

Look for female fitness trainers, teachers, or coaches who focus on women's health and fitness. Working with a female expert who knows your specific goals and problems may give you with tailored direction and support throughout your fitness journey.

8. Participate in mentorship or buddy systems

Seek out mentoring opportunities or buddy networks to connect with more experienced women who can provide direction, advise, and support as you work toward your fitness objectives. A mentor or exercise companion may offer accountability and encouragement along the way.

9. Share Your Journey and Support Others.

 Be open and honest about your fitness journey, experiences, and obstacles. By sharing your story, you create an open and welcoming environment in which other women may share their own experiences and encourage one another.

10. Celebrate Achievements Together

 Celebrate your accomplishments, milestones, and wins with a community of like-minded women. Whether it's achieving a personal fitness goal, finishing a race, or conquering a difficulty, celebrate one other's accomplishments and encourage one another along the way.

Creating a supportive group of like-minded women may improve your fitness journey, give encouragement and inspiration, and foster long-term connections. Connecting with other women who share your enthusiasm for health and wellness allows you to motivate one another, conquer challenges together, and reach your fitness objectives with confidence and fun.

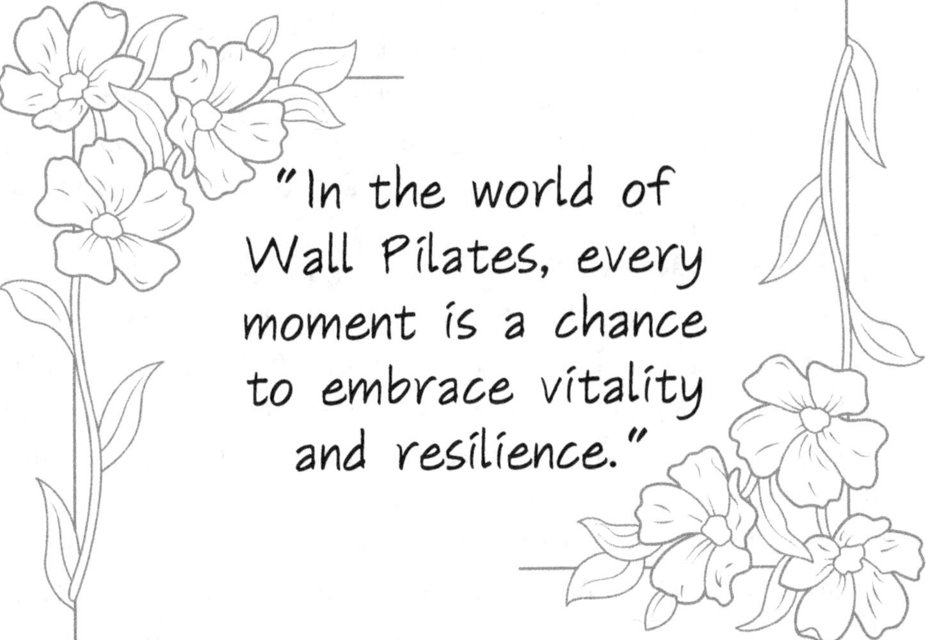

CHAPTER 7

Beyond the Mat

Beyond the mat, adopting holistic well-being entails taking a complete approach to health that goes well beyond the physical practice of yoga. It entails cultivating your entire being—mind, body, and spirit—in order to create a condition of balance, vigor, and fulfillment in life.

At its heart, holistic well-being acknowledges the interdependence of all areas of health and highlights the significance of treating each component in order to reach peak wellness. This holistic approach recognizes that real well-being is more than just the absence of sickness, but also a dynamic condition of thriving in all aspects of life.

Embracing holistic well-being starts with emphasizing self-care techniques that nourish and revitalize the body, mind, and spirit. This may involve engaging in regular physical exercise, eating nutritious meals, getting adequate sleep, and managing stress using mindfulness, meditation, or relaxation techniques.

In addition to physical health, holistic well-being includes mental and emotional well-being, emphasizing the necessity of maintaining a happy attitude, effectively regulating emotions, and building healthy relationships. Developing emotional intelligence, practicing self-compassion, and cultivating meaningful connections with others are all critical components of promoting mental and emotional health.

Furthermore, holistic well-being entails connecting your behaviors and decisions with your beliefs, interests, and life purpose in order to experience a feeling of meaning and fulfillment. This might include making significant objectives, engaging in activities that offer joy and fulfillment, and fostering thankfulness and optimism in daily life.

Beyond individual well-being, holistic well-being acknowledges the interdependence of humans with the environment and the larger society.

It fosters actions that promote environmental sustainability, social justice, and communal well-being, realizing that our own health and well-being are inextricably linked to the health of the world and society as a whole.

In essence, adopting holistic well-being entails a path of self-discovery, self-care, and self-empowerment that touches on all elements of your being. Nurturing your body, mind, and spirit, as well as creating meaningful relationships with others and the environment around you, may lead to a profound sense of completeness, energy, and fulfillment.

Nourishing your Body

Maintaining a good diet and staying hydrated are vital components of overall well-being. Here are some ideas for keeping a healthy diet and staying hydrated:

- Maintain a Balanced Diet - Include nutrient-dense foods from all food categories, such as fruits, vegetables, whole grains, lean protein, and healthy fats. Prioritize healthy, less processed meals over highly processed or sugary alternatives.
- Meal Control: Pay attention to meal proportions to prevent overeating and regulate weight. Use smaller plates, measure portion sizes, and practice mindful eating by paying attention to hunger cues and eating until you're content rather than full.
- Eat fruits and vegetables for vitamins, minerals, fiber, and antioxidants. Aim to fill half of your plate with fruits and vegetables at each meal to improve your overall health and well-being.
- Choose Whole Grains: Choose brown rice, quinoa, oats, whole wheat bread, and pasta over processed grains. Whole grains are high in fiber and minerals, which can help regulate blood sugar and improve digestive health.
- Prioritize Lean Proteins: Include fowl, fish, tofu, beans, lentils, and Greek yogurt in your diet to promote muscle growth, repair, and general health. Limit your intake of processed meat and high-fat animal products.

Consume healthy fats like avocados, nuts, seeds, olive oil, and fatty seafood in your diet. These fats are crucial for brain function, hormone synthesis, and fat-soluble vitamin absorption.

- Stay Hydrated: Drink enough of water throughout the day to promote digestion, circulation, temperature control, and nutrient transfer. Aim to drink at least 8-10 glasses of water every day, or more if you are physically active or in hot weather.
- Limit Sugary Drinks - Avoid sugary beverages including soda, fruit juices, energy drinks, and sweetened teas, which can increase calorie intake and negatively influence health. Instead, choose water, herbal tea, or water flavored with fresh fruits and herbs.
- Plan and prepare meals ahead of time to guarantee healthful selections and avoid harmful convenience foods. Stay on track with your healthy eating goals by batch cooking, meal prepping, and packing snacks to take with you on the move.
- Pay attention to your body's response to different meals and change your diet accordingly. Eat when you're hungry, stop when you're full, and listen to your body's hunger and fullness cues to maintain a balanced relationship with food.

Following these healthy eating and hydration suggestions, you can nourish your body, promote overall well-being, and get the advantages of a balanced and nutritious diet. Remember that little, consistent adjustments over time can result in long-term health and energy.

Managing stress

Managing stress is critical to preserving inner peace and harmony in your life. Including relaxation techniques in your daily routine can help you decrease stress, quiet your mind, and boost overall well-being. Here are some relaxing techniques you might try:

- Deep breathing exercises promote relaxation and alleviate tension. Sit or lie down in a comfortable posture, close your eyes, and inhale slowly and deeply through your nose to fill your lungs with air. Hold for a few seconds before exhaling gently through your mouth, releasing tension and stress with each breath.
- Progressive Muscle Relaxation (PMR) includes progressively tensing and releasing various muscle groups in the body to relieve tension and promote relaxation. Begin by tensing a muscle group, such as your fists or shoulders, for a few seconds before releasing and relaxing entirely. Work your way from head to toe, passing through each muscle group in turn.
- Mindfulness meditation entails focusing on the present moment without judgment. Sit quietly and concentrate on your breath, physiological sensations, or a single item, allowing thoughts and emotions to pass without attachment. Mindfulness meditation can help you reduce stress, develop self-awareness, and find inner peace.
- Gentle yoga and stretching activities can help relieve physical stress, increase flexibility, and promote mental relaxation. To encourage relaxation and stress alleviation, practice yoga positions including child's pose, downward-facing dog, and legs up the wall, with an emphasis on deep breathing and mindful movement.
- Guided imagery is a technique for reducing stress and increasing relaxation by envisioning serene and relaxing landscapes or events. Close your eyes and envision yourself in a peaceful environment, such as a beach, forest, or hilltop. To elicit emotions of calm and inner serenity, concentrate on the sights, sounds, and sensations of your imagined surroundings.
- Tai Chi and Qigong are peaceful mind-body activities that involve slow, flowing motions, deep breathing, and awareness. These ancient techniques encourage relaxation, balance, and harmony in the body and mind, making them useful tools for stress management and general well-being.

- Journaling and expressive writing can help you process emotions, reflect on events, and reduce stress. Set aside time each day to journal about your thoughts, feelings, and experiences, enabling yourself to express and let go of any pent-up emotions or fears
- Spending time in nature can help you connect with nature and find tranquility away from daily stress. To renew your mind and spirit, go for a walk in the park, a hike in the woods, or simply sit outside and take in the sights and sounds of nature.
- Listen to soothing music, nature sounds, or relaxation CDs to encourage relaxation. Experiment with various forms of music or noises to see what connects with you and helps you unwind and relax.
- Hobbies and creative pursuits, including painting, gardening, knitting, or cooking, can provide delight and relaxation. Immersing oneself in enjoyable hobbies can assist to divert your attention away from pressures while also promoting a sense of contentment and wellbeing.

Incorporate these relaxation techniques into your everyday routine to reduce stress, develop inner calm, and cultivate a balanced lifestyle. Experiment with several strategies to see what works best for you, and make self-care and stress management a priority in your overall well-being.

Prioritizing sleep

Prioritizing sleep is critical for general health, well-being, and performance. Adequate rest is crucial for physical healing, cognitive function, emotional equilibrium, and general well-being. Here's why sleep is so essential and how you can make it a priority for your health:

- Sleep promotes physical recovery by allowing the body to heal, restore, and develop. Muscles rebuild themselves, tissues mend, and the immune system strengthens, all of which promote physical recovery and resilience.

- Sleep supports cognitive function, including memory consolidation, learning, problem-solving, and decision-making. Adequate rest improves cognitive performance, creativity, and mental clarity, but sleep deprivation impairs cognitive function and memory recall.
- Emotional Regulation Quality sleep is crucial for regulating emotions and maintaining a stable mood. Adequate rest helps control neurotransmitters and chemicals involved in mood regulation, such as serotonin and cortisol, which lowers the risk of mood disorders including sadness and anxiety.
- Stress Reduction: Sleep reduces cortisol levels and promotes calm. Prioritizing sleep can help you deal with everyday challenges and preserve emotional resilience in difficult times.
- Physical Health: Chronic sleep deprivation increases the risk of obesity, diabetes, heart disease, and immunological dysfunction. Prioritizing sleep can improve overall physical health and lower the risk of chronic illness.
- Quality sleep boosts performance and productivity in personal and professional settings. Adequate rest improves concentration, attention, creativity, problem-solving abilities, and decision-making skills, resulting in higher performance and productivity.
- Sleep is vital for immunological function, regulating immune responses and protecting against diseases. Prioritizing sleep helps boost the immune system and lower the risk of common diseases like colds and the flu.
- Improved Longevity and Quality of Life: Research indicates that getting enough sleep leads to a longer lifetime and higher quality of life. Prioritizing sleep may enhance your general health, energy levels, mood, and vitality, increasing your pleasure of life and longevity.

To prioritize sleep for your well-being, consider the following suggestions:

- Create a regular sleep routine by going to bed and getting up at the same time every day, including weekends.
- Establish a peaceful sleep ritual that signals to your body that it is time to unwind, such as reading, having a warm bath, or practicing relaxation methods.
- Create a restful sleep environment by providing a comfortable mattress, supporting pillows, and a dark, quiet, and cold room.
- Limit your exposure to screens and electronic gadgets before bedtime, since the blue light they generate can interfere with melatonin synthesis and impair sleep.
- Avoid coffee, nicotine, and alcohol close to bedtime since they can impair sleep quality and disturb sleep patterns.
- Prioritize stress-reduction activities like mindfulness, meditation, yoga, or deep breathing exercises to promote relaxation and lessen nocturnal anxiety.
- If you have chronic sleep issues or signs of a sleep disorder, such as insomnia or sleep apnea, see a healthcare expert for an examination and treatment.
- Prioritizing sleep and developing healthy sleep habits may help you maintain your overall well-being, improve your physical and mental health, and reap the countless advantages of restorative sleep for a happier, healthier life.

Living a Vibrant Life

Living a vigorous life entails embracing holistic well-being and achieving harmony in mind, body, and spirit. Pilates is an effective doorway to a healthy you, providing several advantages that contribute to overall vigor and vitality. Here's how Pilates may improve your health and help you live a more active life:

- Pilates promotes core strength, flexibility, muscle balance, and coordination. Regular Pilates practice may help you create a strong, flexible body that moves with ease and elegance, lowering your risk of injury and enhancing lifespan.
- Pilates promotes perfect alignment, posture, and body awareness, resulting in a strong core that supports the spine and maintains good posture. Improved alignment can reduce pain and suffering, increase mobility, and promote overall health.
- Pilates promotes mindfulness and body awareness, resulting in a stronger connection between mind and body. Focused breathing and mindful movement can help you develop a stronger feeling of presence, attention, and inner harmony, lowering tension and increasing relaxation.
- Pilates is a mind-body activity that promotes stress reduction and relaxation. Pilates, which focuses on regulated movements, deep breathing, and conscious awareness, helps relax the nervous system, reduce cortisol levels, and relieve tension and anxiety.
- Regular Pilates exercise can enhance energy, vitality, and quality of life. Pilates boosts physical and mental energy by increasing circulation, oxygenation, and lymphatic flow, leaving you feeling revitalized and renewed.
- Pilates workouts promote functional fitness and enhance daily motions, making them more efficient. Pilates allows you to move more easily, efficiently, and confidently while bending, lifting, reaching, or walking.
- Pilates promotes mindfulness, aware breathing, and inner serenity. Pilates, which focuses on the present moment and connects with your body, may minimize mental chatter, promote self-awareness, and build a deeper feeling of balance and harmony.
- Pilates classes and group sessions offer a chance to interact with others who prioritize their health and well-being.

- Creating a supportive community may boost motivation, accountability, and pleasure of your Pilates practice, increasing your whole experience and instilling a feeling of belonging.
- Pilates promotes personal growth and empowerment. As you grow in your practice, you'll gain more strength, confidence, and resilience, both on and off the mat. Pilates teaches you to listen to your body, trust yourself, and accept your individual path to health and vitality.

By using Pilates as a gateway to a better you, you may harness the transformational power of mind-body exercise and build a vibrant existence full of vitality, pleasure, and well-being. Whether you're new to Pilates or an experienced practitioner, The advantages of this holistic discipline go well beyond the physical, enhancing all aspects of your life and empowering you to live your best life.

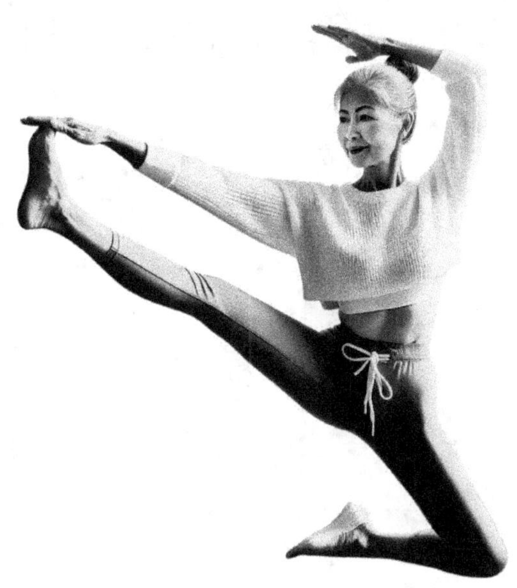

Conclusion

In 'Wall Pilates for Women over 60,' you've unlocked the keys to a vibrant, empowered life. Now, it's time to take that first step toward a stronger, more flexible you. Embrace the transformative power of Wall Pilates and embark on a journey of self-discovery, vitality, and joy. Your body, mind, and spirit will thank you. Are you ready to rewrite the rules of aging and live your best life?

Order your copy today and begin your journey toward strength, balance, and well-being. And as you delve into these pages, I invite you to share your thoughts and experiences.

Your honest review not only helps others discover the benefits of Wall Pilates but also fuels my passion for empowering women on their wellness journeys. **Thank you for joining me on this incredible adventure. Let's thrive together!**

WALL PILATES PROGRESS TRACKER JOURNAL

Daily exercise	Feeling Before Practice	Feeling After Practice	Goals

"Every rep, every breath, brings you closer to your best self. Keep going, keep growing."

WALL PILATES PROGRESS TRACKER JOURNAL

Date: ....

Daily exercise	Feeling Before Practice	Feeling After Practice	Goals

"Every rep, every breath, brings you closer to your best self. Keep going, keep growing."

WALL PILATES PROGRESS TRACKER JOURNAL

Date :...........................

Daily exercise	Feeling Before Practice	Feeling After Practice	Goals

"Every rep, every breath, brings you closer to your best self. Keep going, keep growing."

WALL PILATES PROGRESS TRACKER JOURNAL

Date:..........................

Daily exercise	Feeling Before Practice	Feeling After Practice	Goals

"Every rep, every breath, brings you closer to your best self. Keep going, keep growing."

WALL PILATES PROGRESS TRACKER JOURNAL

Date:.............................

Daily exercise	Feeling Before Practice	Feeling After Practice	Goals

"Every rep, every breath, brings you closer to your best self. Keep going, keep growing."

WALL PILATES PROGRESS TRACKER JOURNAL

Date: ....

Daily exercise	Feeling Before Practice	Feeling After Practice	Goals

"Every rep, every breath, brings you closer to your best self. Keep going, keep growing."

WALL PILATES PROGRESS TRACKER JOURNAL

Date: ....

Daily exercise	Feeling Before Practice	Feeling After Practice	Goals

"Every rep, every breath, brings you closer to your best self. Keep going, keep growing."

WALL PILATES PROGRESS TRACKER JOURNAL

Date:............................

Daily exercise	Feeling Before Practice	Feeling After Practice	Goals

"Every rep, every breath, brings you closer to your best self. Keep going, keep growing."

WALL PILATES PROGRESS TRACKER JOURNAL

Date:.................................

Daily exercise	Feeling Before Practice	Feeling After Practice	Goals

"Every rep, every breath, brings you closer to your best self. Keep going, keep growing."

WALL PILATES PROGRESS TRACKER JOURNAL

Date: ....

Daily exercise	Feeling Before Practice	Feeling After Practice	Goals

"Every rep, every breath, brings you closer to your best self. Keep going, keep growing."

WALL PILATES PROGRESS TRACKER JOURNAL

Date:..............................

Daily exercise	Feeling Before Practice	Feeling After Practice	Goals

"Every rep, every breath, brings you closer to your best self. Keep going, keep growing."

WALL PILATES PROGRESS TRACKER JOURNAL

Date:..............................

Daily exercise	Feeling Before Practice	Feeling After Practice	Goals

"Every rep, every breath, brings you closer to your best self. Keep going, keep growing."

WALL PILATES PROGRESS TRACKER JOURNAL

Date:...........................

Daily exercise	Feeling Before Practice	Feeling After Practice	Goals

"Every rep, every breath, brings you closer to your best self. Keep going, keep growing."

WALL PILATES PROGRESS TRACKER JOURNAL

Date: ....

Daily exercise	Feeling Before Practice	Feeling After Practice	Goals

"Every rep, every breath, brings you closer to your best self. Keep going, keep growing."

WALL PILATES PROGRESS TRACKER JOURNAL

Date:................................

Daily exercise	Feeling Before Practice	Feeling After Practice	Goals

"Every rep, every breath, brings you closer to your best self. Keep going, keep growing."

WALL PILATES PROGRESS TRACKER JOURNAL

Date:............................

Daily exercise	Feeling Before Practice	Feeling After Practice	Goals

"Every rep, every breath, brings you closer to your best self. Keep going, keep growing."

WALL PILATES PROGRESS TRACKER JOURNAL

Date: ....

Daily exercise	Feeling Before Practice	Feeling After Practice	Goals

"Every rep, every breath, brings you closer to your best self. Keep going, keep growing."

WALL PILATES PROGRESS TRACKER JOURNAL

Date:...................................

Daily exercise	Feeling Before Practice	Feeling After Practice	Goals

"Every rep, every breath, brings you closer to your best self. Keep going, keep growing."

WALL PILATES PROGRESS TRACKER JOURNAL

$\mathcal{D}$ate:................................

Daily exercise	Feeling Before Practice	Feeling After Practice	Goals

"Every rep, every breath, brings you closer to your best self. Keep going, keep growing."

WALL PILATES PROGRESS TRACKER JOURNAL

Date:...............................

Daily exercise	Feeling Before Practice	Feeling After Practice	Goals

"Every rep, every breath, brings you closer to your best self. Keep going, keep growing."

WALL PILATES PROGRESS TRACKER JOURNAL

Date: ....

Daily exercise	Feeling Before Practice	Feeling After Practice	Goals

WALL PILATES PROGRESS TRACKER JOURNAL

Date:................................

Daily exercise	Feeling Before Practice	Feeling After Practice	Goals

"Every rep, every breath, brings you closer to your best self. Keep going, keep growing."

WALL PILATES PROGRESS TRACKER JOURNAL

Date:................................

Daily exercise	Feeling Before Practice	Feeling After Practice	Goals

"Every rep, every breath, brings you closer to your best self. Keep going, keep growing."